5 INGREDIENTS OR LESS PLATED COOKBOOK:
(Quick & Easy Cooking)

Recipes to go for ready meals, super easy,
Healthy & Delicious Smart Point Recipes
For Smart and Busy people
Learn in 5min or Less.

LAURA W. GARDNER

Copyright

Disclaimer

The information provided in the "5 ingredients or Less Plated Cookbook 2024" is for General informational purposes only. Although every attempt has been made to offer accurate and Current information, the publisher and author disclaim all explicit and implied warranties and representations on the availability, correctness, appropriateness, completeness, and reliability of the material included within.

The author and publisher disclaim any liability for any loss or damage arising from reliance on the information provided on the cookbook.
Readers are encouraged to consult with a healthcare professional or a qualified nutritionist for individualized advice regarding their dietary choices.

Any reliance you place on the information in this Cookbook is strictly at your own risk. The author and publisher will not be liable for any losses and damages in connection with the use of this Cookbook

About the author

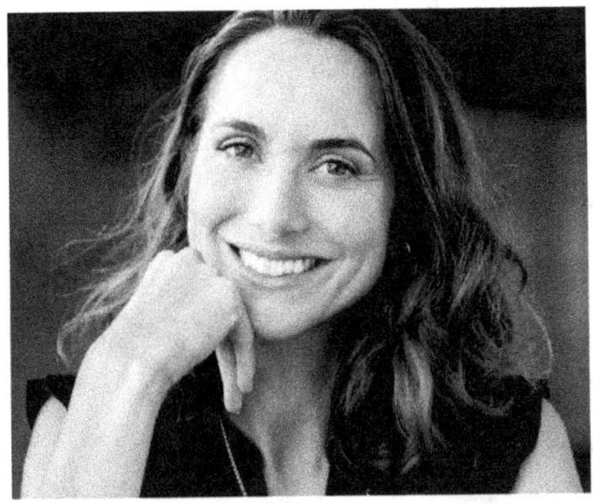

Welcome to the world of savory, wholesome, and quick cooking, all under Laura W. Gardner's culinary tutelage. As a seasoned chef and fervent supporter of healthy living, Laura has devoted her culinary career to developing quick, wholesome, and mouthwatering recipes that stimulate the senses while

simultaneously providing nourishment to the body.

Laura's passion for cooking started at a young age, sparked by the diverse range of flavors found in her ethnic background. She was raised in a home that valued healthful ingredients and home-cooked meals, and she was taught the idea of providing the body with foods high in nutrients. Her subsequent efforts in the field of healthy eating were made possible by this foundation.

Laura sought formal studies in nutrition and culinary sciences because she was very interested in investigating the relationship between health and culinary arts. Equipped with erudition and a fervor for healthful cooking, she set out to reinterpret the notion that nutritious cuisine has to be boring and time-consuming.

Laura blends a creative flair with a thorough awareness of nutrition in her culinary

creations. Her meals serve as evidence that preparing healthy food doesn't have to involve spending a lot of time in the kitchen or compromising flavor. Laura's recipes suit a wide range of tastes and lifestyles, whether you're a working professional, a parent on the go, or someone just looking for a tasty and nutritious supper.

In addition to sharing her delicious recipes, Laura offers advice on sustainable living, thoughtful eating, and the delight that comes from appreciating each bite. Her cooking philosophy is holistic, taking into account how one's dietary decisions affect the environment as well as the human.

Laura is a culinary influencer who uses her blog, cooking classes, and social media to interact with her community. Aspiring cooks are encouraged to go on a journey with her towards a happier and healthier living via the lone's dietary decisions affect the environment as well as the human.

Laura is a culinary influencer who uses her blog, cooking classes, and social media to interact with her community. Aspiring cooks are encouraged to go on a journey with her towards a happier and healthier living via the joy of cooking, thanks to her kind and approachable personality. regardless of your experience level as a home cook. Discover a world of quick, wholesome, and delicious dishes that will change the way you view food and the way you interact with the meals that give you energy. Prepare to go on a gastronomic adventure with Laura W. Gardner that feeds your body and soul.

Contents

INTRODUCTION

Hello there, fellow avid eaters! Life's moving at a lightning pace, and we get it, you want meals that are not just fast but also good for you and seriously tasty. Well, you're in for a treat because we're diving into the world of Fast, Healthy, and Tasty Recipes, where deliciousness meets efficiency!

Picture this: Mouthwatering dishes that won't have you spending hours in the kitchen but will still make your taste buds do a happy dance. We believe that fast food doesn't have to be synonymous with unhealthy, and healthy meals don't have to be bland or boring. Our recipes are like culinary superheroes, saving you time and delivering a flavor-packed punch.

Who's behind this culinary adventure? It's us, a bunch of food lovers who understand the struggles of daily life. Whether you're a workaholic, a parent on the go, or just someone who craves good food without the fuss, we've got you covered. These recipes are more than just quick fixes, they're a celebration of flavors that will make you forget you're eating something good for you.

So, get ready to ditch the notion that fast equals junk and join us on a journey where every meal is a happy compromise between time constraints and the desire for something seriously tasty. We're flipping the script on what it means to cook in a hurry, because in our world, fast, healthy, and tasty aren't mutually exclusive, they're the perfect recipe for a satisfying meal. Let's dive in and make cooking a joyous experience where every bite is a nod to the sweet spot where health meets flavor!

This Cookbook is more than just a list of recipes that people can use as a resource for culinary experimentation and explorations.
They are semi-autobiographical in that this book becomes an immortalization of Laura W. Gardner turning points when she selects recollections from childhood, times when the food is not only eaten but also celebrated. The cookbook offers food and memories to people who might enjoy them as well.

This book has quick, inexpensive, and healthful dishes that will appeal to all types of cooks. Most of the recipes only take ten to fifteen minutes to prepare.
This Cookbook is more than just a list of recipes that people can use as a resource for culinary experimentation and explorations.
They are semi-autobiographical in that this book becomes an immortalization of Laura W. Gardner turning points when she selects recollections from childhood, times when the food is not only eaten but also celebrated. The cookbook offers food and memories to people who might enjoy them as well.
This book has quick, inexpensive, and healthful dishes that will appeal to all types of cooks. Most of the recipes only take five to fifteen minutes to prepare.

How I came to understand what I meant by healthy eating

Eating healthier is a popular New Year's Resolution that many people make every year. But what does that mean? It all relies on what your body needs to achieve your specific objectives.

Eating healthily can take many forms, and determining what that means for you may take some time.

For me, it began with examining the effects of the foods I chose on my body.

Many people choose drastic measures, they abruptly decide to become vegans only eating quinoa, kale, and chia seeds, or they resolve to become 100% gluten-free. Those methods may be in style, but they're probably not long-term.

Each person has different dietary needs or requirements. It depends on a plethora of factors, including lifestyle and health objectives. To get it right, observation and practice are required.

NOT EVERY BODY FUNCTIONS THE SAME.

It's no secret that the media adores discussing trendy eating plans. However, no diet or significant lifestyle adjustment will be effective for everyone. Eating paleo or monitoring macros may work well for certain people, but there isn't a single, universally applicable approach.

To be clear, there is a huge difference between "dieting" and "eating healthily." The difference between "healthy" and "skinny" has been a major realization for me and I believe for many women as well. You can eat the things you enjoy and still be healthy. Seldom are restrictions the path to pleasure (or health)!

Having said that, I've really enjoyed discovering how to "healthify" my greatest urges.

I've roasted a good number of sweet potatoes, created buckets of banana ice cream, and discovered that flavoring food with a variety of spices and herbs rather than just salt is possible. My meals taste wonderful and often make me feel happy. This encourages me to eat more healthily.

I now eat better meals, but I also see food in a healthy light and adjust my perspective accordingly. I'm more at ease, sleep better, and concentrate better. My meals are something I eagerly anticipate and I never feel bad about eating them.

Remember that eating is about more than just providing your body with nourishment, this year as you set out on your personal health

journey. It's also about having fun. Look for foods that bring you joy and wellness. "Eating healthy" can refer to making decisions that make you happy in addition to your physical health.

You're far more likely to continue with your new routine if you're genuinely enjoying it. Think about how your body reacts to various foods.

If you're like me, you'll discover that loving your body begins with enjoying your food, and when you do, your body is far more inclined to love you in return.

GOING BACK TO THE BASICS: TEN ESSENTIAL INGREDIENTS EVERY KITCHEN NEEDS

for baking, your lighter, more subdued one for sautéing, and your less expensive one for salads.

GARLIC WITH ONIONS

These two flavor-bomb components go into almost every dish (some of us even sneak them into breakfast). And when cooking at home becomes increasingly popular (hey, Covid), garlic and onions can pretty much make any dish better. The cook uses it as a cheat ingredient; just add some to a pan with butter and the family will be drooling.

TOMATOES IN A CAN

Given that they are among the most adaptable pantry staples, it should come as no surprise. Desire some bolognese? Simple. What about cacciatore chicken? You understand. Do you want to try making your own pizza? You have Tom's back.

FLOUR

Whatever the kind, flour is a constant. There is flour out there for every home cook, and they should be in your pantry. Whether it's the "bread-y" kind that works well for handmade bread, spaghetti, and pizza, the finer cake flour to produce those bouncy, delectable delights, or even simply a go-to cheapie to beef up your Sunday night gravy.

PASTA

Italy will come to us if we are unable to travel there. Whatever your preference for

pasta, large, fat rigatoni, long, flat fettuccine, or flamboyant, dramatic farfalle, you should always have a variety on hand. Pasta is a pantry staple that's great for easy midweek meals or as the ideal side dish for a slow-cooked ragu during the weekend.

Every type of cheese, brie, cheddar, goat's, feta, blue, or cream, has a special place in our hearts and refrigerators. They enhance the flavor of cakes, thicken sauces, add oozey goodness in between bread slices, dress up salads, and can even be consumed by the wedge (load). We welcome this indispensable cooking item with open arms.

SPICES
Even if your dish is already excellent, adding a dash of spice might make it even better. To give an additional flavor dimension to meat, fish, or poultry, sprinkle spices on top and mix them into sauces.

VINEGAR
All vinegars are beneficial in the kitchen, especially for marinades, dressings, and pickling; this includes balsamic, rice, apple cider, malt, cane, and white vinegars. Sharp flavors can cut through cheese, temper sweetness in salads, and enhance meat flavors.

RICE
When you have a gorgeous sauce, it should be paired with equally gorgeous fluffy rice. This culinary essential is a crowd-pleaser for the whole family and the foundation of any casserole, stir-fry, or curry. Of course, if you're a real aficionado, you could even prepare a zesty fried rice dish or an exquisite risotto. There are countless options.

Every type of cheese, brie, cheddar, goat's, feta, blue, or cream, has a special place in our hearts and refrigerators. They enhance the flavor of cakes, thicken sauces, add oozey goodness in between bread slices, dress up salads, and can even be consumed by the wedge (load). We welcome this indispensable cooking item with open arms.

SPICES

Even if your dish is already excellent, adding a dash of spice might make it even better. To give an additional flavor dimension to meat, fish, or poultry, sprinkle spices on top and mix them into sauces.

VINEGAR

All vinegars are beneficial in the kitchen, especially for marinades, dressings, and pickling; this includes balsamic, rice, apple cider, malt, cane, and white vinegars. Sharp flavors can cut through cheese, temper sweetness in salads, and enhance meat flavors.

RICE

When you have a gorgeous sauce, it should be paired with equally gorgeous fluffy rice. This culinary essential is a crowd-pleaser for the whole family and the foundation of any casserole, stir-fry, or curry. Of course, if you're a real aficionado, you could even prepare a zesty fried rice dish or an exquisite risotto. There are countless options.

10 Practical Tips to Help You Become a Better Cook:

There will be no hackers, tricks, or magic. Just the facts.

If you've ever tried to locate a single list of universal cooking hacks, tips, rules, or general advice on how to improve or take your cooking to the next level, you know how difficult it is.

You wind up in a sea of clickbait listicles, most of which contain a previously viral kitchen technique, some words from a prominent Food Network star, and a lot of photographs. While all of them are enjoyable and certainly a good way to pass the time, they never provide a firm, honest response to the question "What is important to know to become a better cook?"

The ten ideas you're going to discover aren't your average kitchen hacks. These suggestions will not miraculously transform you into Gordon Ramsay, but they will provide you with a clear picture of what to focus on when preparing your next meal and what culinary skills you need to learn or improve on.

And guess what? Even Gordon Ramsay would most likely agree with everything on this list. So let's get started:

1. Cooking is a skill. Baking Is An Art.

Have you previously heard anything similar? Since the 1960s, this famous quote has been cited in print. Some food professionals disagree, claiming that cooking and baking are both. However, if you lack culinary school instruction and years of restaurant kitchen experience, you should normally adhere to this rule.

What does it imply?
When attempting a new recipe, taste and modify the flavors as you go. Most recipes are only recommendations, and you may either add more spice if you prefer it hot or skip one of the components if you detest it or are allergic to it.
Cooking is a subjective and forgiving art.

You may enjoy the Scoville heat of 500,000 and up in chocolate habanero peppers, but

Most people will not appreciate such a severe kick to their taste receptors and will not consume those peppers unless there is a monetary award or they have lost some harsh bet.
So just taste as you cook, taste your dish at each stage, and adjust as needed. With practice, patience, and a broad understanding of different spices and flavor combinations, you should be able to save any dish before it reaches the dinner table.

spices and flavor combinations, you should be able to save any dish before it reaches the dinner table.

When it comes to baking, it's a very different story. All baking recipes provide accurate amounts of ingredients, detailed stages, and strategies, and if you follow them exactly, you will get the desired result.
See! It's exactly like a science experiment. It is accurate and reproducible on a consistent basis. Try modifying a souffle recipe to better

suit your taste palate, and whatever you end up with will no longer be recognized as a souffle. It will be something, but it will not be a souffle.

If you are a true home baker who has mastered multiple ways, then go ahead and take your chances and experiment.Even yet, there will be times when your baking endeavors will fail spectacularly.

When cooking, always taste your food. As you continue, adjust the tastes.
Baked goods recipes must be followed properly. It's also a good idea to use a kitchen scale.

2. Learn What Umami Is and How to Use It in Savory Recipes

If the phrase 'umami' when describing flavor is unknown to you, stop reading immediately and google it.

'The fifth flavor is umami'. Sweet, sour, salty, bitter, and umami are all flavors. A Japanese scientist coined the name, and it was only in the 1980s that it was formally recognized as the fifth (and most mystical) flavor. Umami, loosely translated as "pleasantly savory," is difficult to describe.

Can you describe what "salty" tastes like in words? Exactly! Salty tastes like, well, salty... and umami tastes delicious. It adds fleeting richness to all flavors and makes your savory recipes more appealing. Amazing.

The problematic issue is that there is no specific store where you can buy umami for your Sunday roast. You may be wondering where I got this umami stuff.

The mystical fifth flavor is obtained by employing so-called 'umami agents' in your cookery. To offer you some examples: Cured meats, anchovies, kimchi, and sun-dried tomatoes, with fish and oyster sauce.

3. Understand Your Salts and Keep It Kosher

Have you ever read a recipe that specifically instructs you to use Kosher salt? Ever pondered why this is the case?

Kosher salt has nothing to do with dietary requirements. It is a coarse-grained salt that does not include iodine and was originally intended for koshering meat (removing all the blood from it).

Many recipes now recommend using Kosher salt because salt without iodine simply tastes better. Its large, light flakes do not dissolve right away and help to evenly salt your meals during the cooking process.

As a general guideline, use Kosher salt for cooking and baking, and sea salt to season your foods. Forget table salt, which contains iodine and other chemicals.

4. Recognize the Hydrogen's Power or the Importance of Acid

You know when you taste something and think to yourself, "Something is missing..." The missing element you're referring to is acid 9 times out of 10.

In cooking, acidity (or pH level) is critical. In culinary school, there is a whole subject dedicated to acid and base in food science. But there isn't time for that. Remember that

acid enhances flavors, adds depth, and helps put everything into harmony.

Wine and vinegar are essential components for soups, sauces, vinaigrettes, and deglazing (more on deglazing later). When a recipe calls for a dash or a splash, don't forget or neglect these two; they make a difference.

Citrus: Lemons, limes, oranges, and other citrus fruits are known for reducing the fishiness in seafood and brightening grilled chicken and many cooked vegetables. A little citrus juice or zest can make a big difference in any dish.

Sour cream, buttermilk, crème fraîche, or yogurt add light and fresh accents to savory recipes and keep baked goods moist and soft. They also make fantastic sauces with garlic and herbs.

Coffee is acidic, which you may be startled to find. Fresh coffee grounds, on the other hand, are used as rubs for roasted or grilled meats. And it is coffee's acidity that is responsible for all coffee-related food hacks.

It makes a difference to add a little coffee to your soup, chili, or stew. And incorporating freshly brewed coffee into chocolate cake batter is a well-known strategy to enhance the chocolate flavor.

5. Brine the meat

There's a proven approach to avoid dry, chewy, or flavorless pork chops, chicken breast, or turkey. Simply brine the lean slices of beef before cooking.

Brining tenderizes the meat and allows it to retain all of its juices when cooked. Food science enchantment!

Don't be concerned that brining is a difficult process requiring difficult-to-find ingredients. All you need is water, salt, and a little time.

If you're cooking a whole bird, soak it in the salty water solution for at least 12 hours. If it's only pork chops or chicken breast, you don't need to cook it for so long. 1 Brine for one hour per pound, generally speaking.

For a normal brine solution, dissolve one cup of Kosher salt in one gallon of water.
There are many nicer brine alternatives available, but this basic one works like magic every time.

6. Understand Your Heat

Whatever food you choose to prepare, the required heat level will always be specified in the cooking directions. There are four heat levels to be aware of:

This is the setting for simmering.

Medium heat is ideal for quick simmering or moderate cooking. For example, when you wish to soften your vegetables.

Most of your cooking will most likely be done over medium-high heat. This is where you will conduct the most of your frying, browning, and sautéing. It still allows you to cook quickly without burning it. You use it to cook your food from start to finish.

High heat: you begin or end your cooking process on high heat. You don't use it all the way through to cook your food. High heat is used to sear meat, sauté vegetables, and thicken sauces.

The recipe will almost certainly require you to adjust the heat level once or twice, and you should. Don't use the same degree of heat from beginning to end.

7. Understand Your Frying Pans

And here we are again, with a conundrum and a plethora of contradictory online pages.

But first and foremost. When it comes to pans, one tip to remember is "don't invest in cheap." These are your primary tools, therefore it makes sense to invest in a few high-quality ones.

And honestly, you only require a few.

When you see headlines like "Toss your nonstick and use cast iron for everything" or "You can cook anything in your cast iron skillet," it's easy to become confused.

The truth is that cast iron skillets are incredible. If you're fortunate enough to acquire one from your mother or grandmother, it should be one of your primary kitchen equipment. However, you

should not throw away the non-stick pan. They are not in competition; they are simply different.

I'll explain; it's best to have at least four pans in your kitchen: a nonstick pan, a stainless steel pan, and a couple of cast iron skillets.

Do I really need two cast iron skillets?" And what can a stainless steel pan achieve that the other two cannot? There are a few things to think about:

Remember that the cast-iron surface absorbs flavors.

A cast-iron skillet has a porous surface that absorbs the tastes of the food cooked in it, especially if it's fresh and new. Even an heirloom skillet that has been seasoned multiple times is susceptible to retaining flavor. It makes even more sense given that

you shouldn't wash them with normal dish soap. Assume you just finished a delicious short rib roast in it for Friday dinner and intend to make the renowned iron
 Saturday skillet cookies... This is probably not the finest idea.

This is why it would be good to have two of them, one for sweet and the other for savory.

Consider the temperature (rule 6)

Cast iron skillets are fantastic for high-heat cooking. They're your go-to for the greatest sear, browning, and crunchy crust. Their superior heat retention poses an issue for delicate meat and fish. This is why we also require the stainless steel pan. To put it simply:

Cast iron skillets are ideal for any cuisine that requires high heat and is not too delicate.

Stainless steel pan: ensures even medium-high and high-heat cooking.

When you want the crunch and a great seer but don't want it to stick or fall apart, use it for more delicate items like fish, shrimp, and veggies.

In a nonstick pan, use low to medium heat. Perfect for fluffy omelets, delicate crepes, or soft scrambled eggs.

Don't overlook acidity (pH values).

Acidic meals should be cooked in a stainless steel pan. Easy.

Slow-cooking tomato sauces or deglazing with alcohol or vinegar will corrode your cast iron. Over time, acid causes the seasoning on your pan to deteriorate. As a result, some of your foods will eventually taste metallic. It's not a health risk, but it's certainly unpleasant.

Cooking acidic foods in a nonstick pan is never a good idea. It will deteriorate the nonstick coating over time, and in that case, it is not just the taste of your food altering; it is exceedingly hazardous and harmful.

Bonus: Purchase a Dutch Oven as well.

Don't buy on a budget. When cooking in a cast iron skillet, stainless steel pan, or nonstick pan, keep heat, food texture, and acidity in mind. Yes, it is significant.

8. Always deglaze your skillet.

Don't be put off by the word 'deglaze,' although it may sound fancy. Deglazing a hot skillet is as simple as pouring liquid to it. You used to sauté some onions and garlic, sear a piece of meat, or do something else that leaves some wonderful browned bits on the bottom of your pan.

If you're still unsure, check out step-by-step guide to deglazing a pan.

9. Distinct Flavors and Textures Prepare a Well-Balanced Dish

This is perhaps the most difficult to learn, but it is crucial to comprehend.

Think about the pictures that are used to describe recipes or on restaurant menus.

It's always a contrasting blend of "crunchy coating with tender and juicy...", "flavorful yet tender...", "salty with notes of sweetness...", "smoky with spicy..."

Even some of your favorite flavors that you don't think about very often are diametrically opposed (sweet and sour chicken, anyone?).

This is not something you should try to study; rather, it is more about paying attention to contrasting flavors and textures and making a mental note of which ones work best together.

Does it make sense to apply the "live in the moment" philosophy to food? Simply be aware of what your taste senses are attempting to tell you. You will ultimately 'feel' it.

10. Experiment with New Things

Last but not least, keep curious and don't be afraid to take risks (though perhaps not while baking). Try new dishes, eat at new restaurants, and learn about new cuisines.

"If you don't know what 'delicious' is supposed to taste like, how can you cook anything delicious?" says my grandmother, who is an exceptional cook. That is really true!

Consume more of everything, try different flavors, and learn more about what good food should taste like.

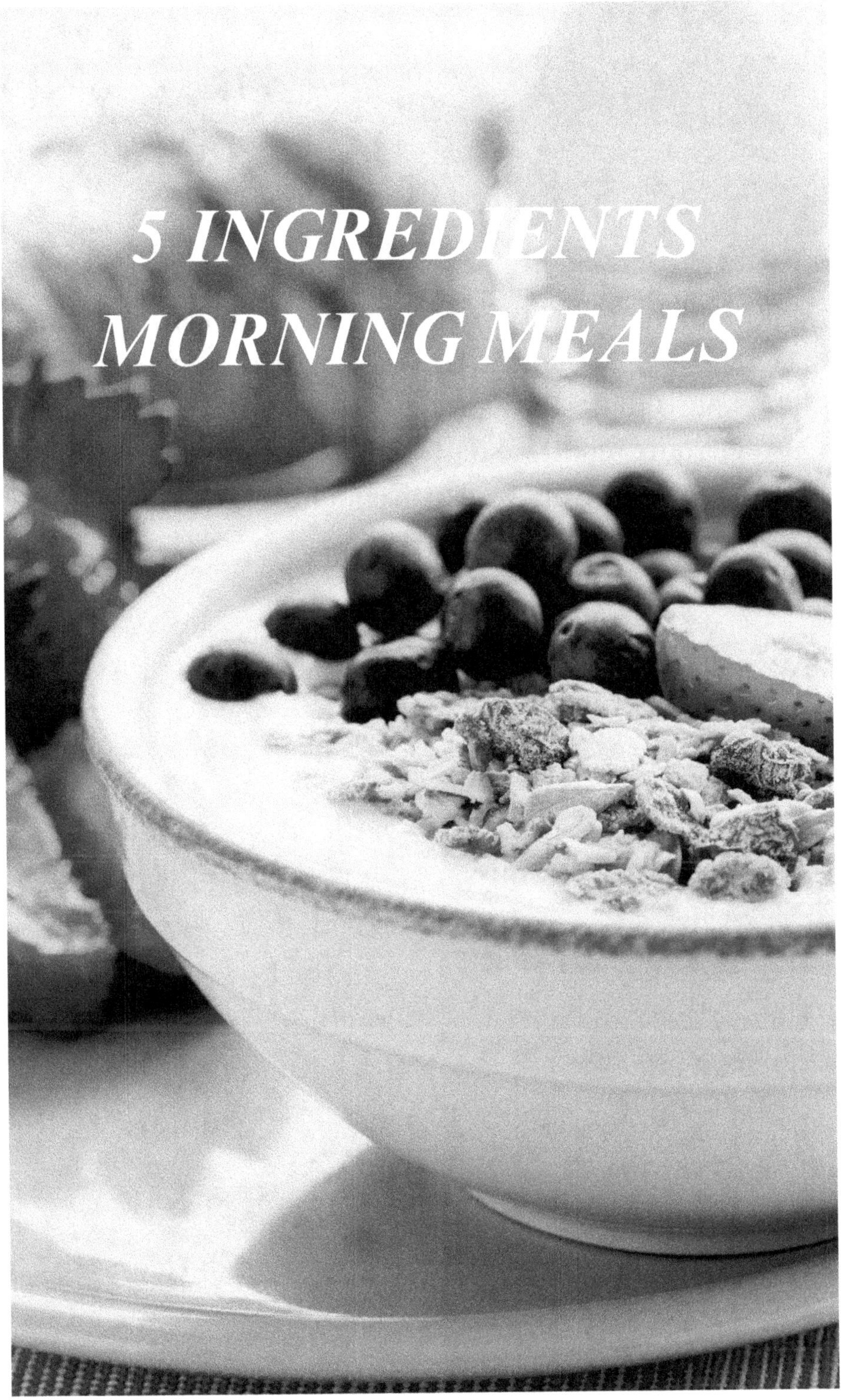

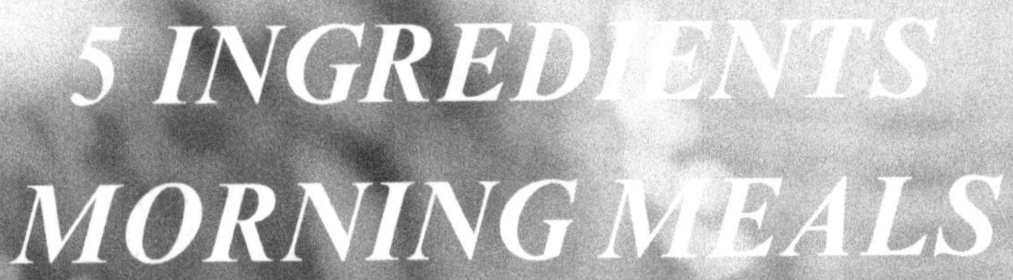
5 INGREDIENTS
MORNING MEALS

POTATO WAFFLES #5FIX

5-Ingredient Fix. From the first bite, these delicious stacked potato waffles with gooey Mexican eggs will tantalize your taste buds. Their 'flavorful fiesta' bursts inside your mouth. Your family and friends will be requesting this filling dish frequently because it is so tasty and irresistible."

INGREDIENTS

Just Potatoes® Shredded Hash Browns, 2 cups
One cup of chunky, thick salsa
Eight sizable eggs
Two cups of mixed Mexican cheese
8 tablespoons finely chopped cilantro

DIRECTIONS

Preheat a nonstick waffle iron and season per the instructions provided by the manufacturer.

Combine potatoes, 1/3 cup salsa, and 2 beaten eggs in a medium-sized bowl.

Combine everything together.Pour mixture into heated waffle iron, ensuring borders are equally distributed. After covering and cooking the potato waffles for at least 15 to 20 minutes, they should be crispy, brown, and done.

Beat the remaining six eggs in a medium-sized bowl. Blend in 1/3 cup of salsa by mixing thoroughly.

With a nonstick skillet, preheat it to medium. Pour the egg mixture into a heated skillet, then scramble the eggs by mixing and stirring with a spatula and scraping the bottom of the pan. Stir and simmer for another minute after adding one cup of cheese.

Stir and simmer for another minute after adding one cup of cheese.

When the cheese appears melted and the eggs reach the correct consistency, remove from the fire.

Avoid overcooking. Scatter the leftover cup of cheese evenly on top of the eggs. When the potato waffles are done cooking, cover and keep warm.

After the waffles are finished, cut them into fours according to the waffle maker's compartment lines. Arrange each waffle quarterwise on a plate. Arrange the melted

Place a dollop of Salsa in the middle of the cheese and continue with the remaining plates. Top each plate with two Tablespoons of freshly chopped cilantro.

Warm up the food.
Makes 4 substantial, delectable servings.
Serve extra salsa in a bowl if you'd like.

PANEAS WITH OATMEAL COTTAGE CHEESE

INGREDIENTS

A half-cup each of oats and cottage cheese
One teaspoon of vanilla four egg whites

DIRECTION

In a blender, combine all the ingredients.
Coat a skillet with cooking spray and fry a few little pancakes at a time, similar to "silver dollar" pancakes. Add your preferred pancake topping on top!

BERRY & PEANUT BUTTER WAFFLE SANDWICH

The foundation for a filling meal that tastes just like a traditional peanut butter and jelly sandwich is made from whole-grain freezer waffles. To add texture, we use crunchy peanut butter, but if you'd rather, you may use creamy. If you can't find fresh berries, you may use frozen ones; defrost them in the microwave for about 30 seconds in a small bowl before adding them to the sandwich.

INGREDIENTS

1 toasted whole-wheat freezer waffle

One tablespoon of natural, crunchy peanut butter

quarter of a cup of fresh mixed berries, including blackberries, strawberries, and raspberries

A tsp of honey

INSTRUCTIONS

Cut the waffle in half lengthwise. Cover half of the other with peanut butter.
The berries should be placed in a small basin

and crushed with a fork.

Spread over the peanut butter layer, followed by a honey drizzle. Place the remaining waffle half on top.

DIY YOGURT

"I've had this recipe for almost thirty years, but I honestly can't recall where I found it." Using this method was my usual practice as I never owned a "yogurt maker". This recipe yields an unexpectedly delicious "plain" yogurt.

**Note: You can use your homemade plain yogurt as the starter for subsequent batches after you prepare your first batch of homemade yogurt.
**Cook/prep durations do not include the 4 hour setting time or the 8 hour chilling period."

INGREDIENTS

1/2 gallon of whole milk (skim or low-fat milk can also be used)
1/2 cup yogurt starter (store-bought plain yogurt will work as long as it has "live cultures") or 1/2 cup mahdzoon

DIRECTIONS

After bringing milk to a gentle boil, let it cool. Just cold enough (approximately 120°F) so that you can't bite your finger.

Transfer the heated milk into a glass or Pyrex bowl, then include the Mahdzoon starter (or store-purchased "live culture" plain yogurt).

Stir in the starter and thoroughly mix, then cover.

To keep the temperature consistent, completely cover the bowl with towels on both the top and bottom.

Cover and leave at room temperature for three to four hours, or until the mahdzoon sets.

Let cool for eight hours before serving.

Store in the refrigerator to preserve.

Before serving, you can optionally add a spoonful or two of jam or preserves and a small amount of vanilla.

BOX OF CEREAL BREAKFAST SUNDAE

INGREDIENTS

1/2 cup berries, at your discretion

1/2 cup yogurt, vanilla or any other flavor you want

1/4 cup cereal (you can choose low-fat cinnamon granolas, cheerios, or crispy rice, again).

DIRECTIONS

First layer the fruit, then the yogurt, and finally the cereal in a glass or parfait dish.

To finish, repeat twice more and top with a layer of cereal.

Add your preferred strawberry or fruit on top, if you'd like.

EVERYTHING BAGELS AVOCADO TOAST

INGREDIENTS

¼ medium avocado, mashed

One toasted slice of whole-grain bread

Two tsp of the everything bagel spice

A pinch of crumbly sea salt (like Maldon)

GUIDELINES

Toast with avocado spread on it. Add salt and spice on top.

For those who enjoy sweetness, add a spoonful of honey.

PEANUT BUTTER AND CHIA BERRY JAM ENGLISH

INGREDIENTS

Muffins

½ cup frozen mixed berries without added sugar

Two tsp of chia seeds

Two tsp natural peanut butter

One toasted whole-wheat English muffin

GUIDELINES

Place berries in a medium bowl that is safe to microwave for 30 seconds.

mix, then microwave for an additional 30 seconds. Add the chia seeds and stir.

On the English muffin, spread peanut butter. Add the berry-chia mixture on top.

BERRY-MINT KEFIR

INGREDIENTS

One cup of plain, low-fat kefir (see Tip)

One cup of frozen mixed berries

Half a cup of orange juice

One or two tablespoons of fresh mint

One tablespoon of honey

GUIDELINES

In a blender, combine kefir, berries, juice, honey, and mint to taste. Process till everything is smooth. (The smoothies can be frozen for up to three months or refrigerated for up to one day.)

Advice: Most stores carry drinkable yogurt called kefir in their dairy area.

QUICK CHEESE & EGG "BAKE"

Discover how to prepare eggs in the microwave for a tasty and speedy meal. Cheddar cheese and spinach give these eggs even more substance.

INGREDIENTS

one cup of finely chopped spinach

Two big eggs

One tsp of milk

Two tablespoons of cheddar cheese, shredded

One warmed corn tortilla

GUIDELINES

Apply cooking spray to an 8-ounce ramekin. Include spinach. Turn the heat to High and let it wilt for about 30 seconds. Top with cracked eggs, milk drizzle, and salt & pepper to taste. Add some cheese on top of it. For approximately two minutes, cook the eggs on High until they are set. Accompany with a tortilla.

RICOTTA-BERRY CREPES

INGREDIENTS

1 whole-wheat crepe

Two tsp fat-free ricotta cheese

¼ cup berries

One tablespoon of honey

GUIDELINES

Spread ricotta over the crepe. Top with berries. For up to a month, fold, wrap in foil, and freeze.

To consume and reheat: Remove the wrapping and zap for one minute at a time until well heated. Garnish with honey, if you prefer

WHOLE WHEAT BAGEL WITH PEANUT BUTTER

INGREDIENTS

One tiny bagel made entirely of whole wheat

One tablespoon of genuine, creamy peanut butter

One big orange

INSTRUCTIONS

Toast a bagel. Dip bagel halves in peanut butter. Serve with an orange.

CHORIZO & EGGS WRAPS

INGREDIENTS

Twelve ounces of new chorizo
Six big eggs
two tsp 2% milk
One cup of cheddar cheese, shredded
Six eight-inch flour tortillas, reheated
Extra toppings at your discretion: Salsa, thinly sliced green onions, and freshly minced cilantro

GUIDELINES

Take the chorizo out of the casings. Cook the chorizo in a large cast-iron skillet or other heavy skillet over medium heat for 6 to 8 minutes, or until it is cooked through and crumbles. Empty and put back into the pan. Whisk together the eggs and milk in a small bowl. To the chorizo, add the egg mixture.

Cook and stir until no liquid egg is left in the eggs and they have thickened. Add cheese and stir. Fill the center of each tortilla with 1/2 cup of the egg mixture.

Add the desired toppings. Roll up the tortilla by folding its edges and bottom over the filling.

PANCAKES WITH CINNAMON APPLESAUCE

INGREDIENTS

1 cup fully prepared buttermilk pancake mix

1 teaspoon cinnamon powder

1 cup cinnamon chunky applesauce

14 cup of water

Butter and maple syrup

DIRECTIONS

Combine the pancake mix and cinnamon in a mixing bowl.

Stir in the applesauce and water until just moistened.

Pour batter by 1/4 cupfuls onto a hot griddle that has been oiled turn when bubbles appear on top. Cook till golden brown on the second side. Serve along with syrup and butter.

CUBAN BREAKFAST SANDWICHES

INGREDIENTS

1 pound of Cuban or French bread 4 big eggs

16 firm salami slices, thinly cut

8 deli ham slices 8 swiss cheese slices

DIRECTIONS

Cut the bread in half lengthwise and then into four pieces. Fry eggs in a large skillet covered with cooking spray until the yolks are firm.

Arrange cheese, ham, salami, and egg on the bottom of the bread, then replace the tops. Cook on a panini press or indoor grill for 2 minutes, or until the cheese has melted and the bread has gotten brown.

CHERRY-ALMOND OATMEAL

Do you want breakfast ready for you when the sun rises? If so, give this hot cereal a try. Simply put the ingredients in the slow cooker and turn it on before going to bed. Enjoy a nutritious, warm, and filling breakfast.

INGREDIENTS

4 cups vanilla flavored almond milk
1 cup rolled oats 1 cup dried cherries
1/3 cup brown sugar, packed
1/2 teaspoon salt
1/2 teaspoon cinnamon powder

DIRECTIONS

Combine all ingredients in a 3-quart slow cooker covered with cooking spray.

Cook, covered, over low heat for 7-8 hours, or until oats are soft.

Mix it thoroughly before serving. Serve with more milk if desired.

YOGURT & HONEY FRUIT CUPS

INGREDIENTS

4 1/2 cups fresh fruit, sliced up (pears, apples, bananas, grapes, etc.)
3/4 cup yogurt (mandarin orange, vanilla, or lemon)
1 teaspoon honey
1/4 teaspoon almond extract 1/2 teaspoon grated orange zest

DIRECTIONS

Divide the fruit into six individual serving dishes. Drizzle the fruit with yogurt, honey, orange zest, and extract.

CHORIZO SALSA OMELET

INGREDIENTS

1 tablespoon butter
3 large eggs,
3 tablespoons water,
1/8 teaspoon salt,
and 1/4 cup cooked chorizo or sausage
2 heaping teaspoons chunky salsa

DIRECTIONS

Melt butter in a small nonstick skillet over medium-high heat. Beat the eggs, water, salt, and pepper together.

Pour the egg mixture onto the skillet (the mixture should solidify instantly around the sides).

As the eggs set, press the cooked edge toward the center, allowing the uncooked half to flow beneath. When the eggs are done, put the chorizo and salsa on one side and fold the other side over the filling.

Spoon the omelet onto a serving dish.

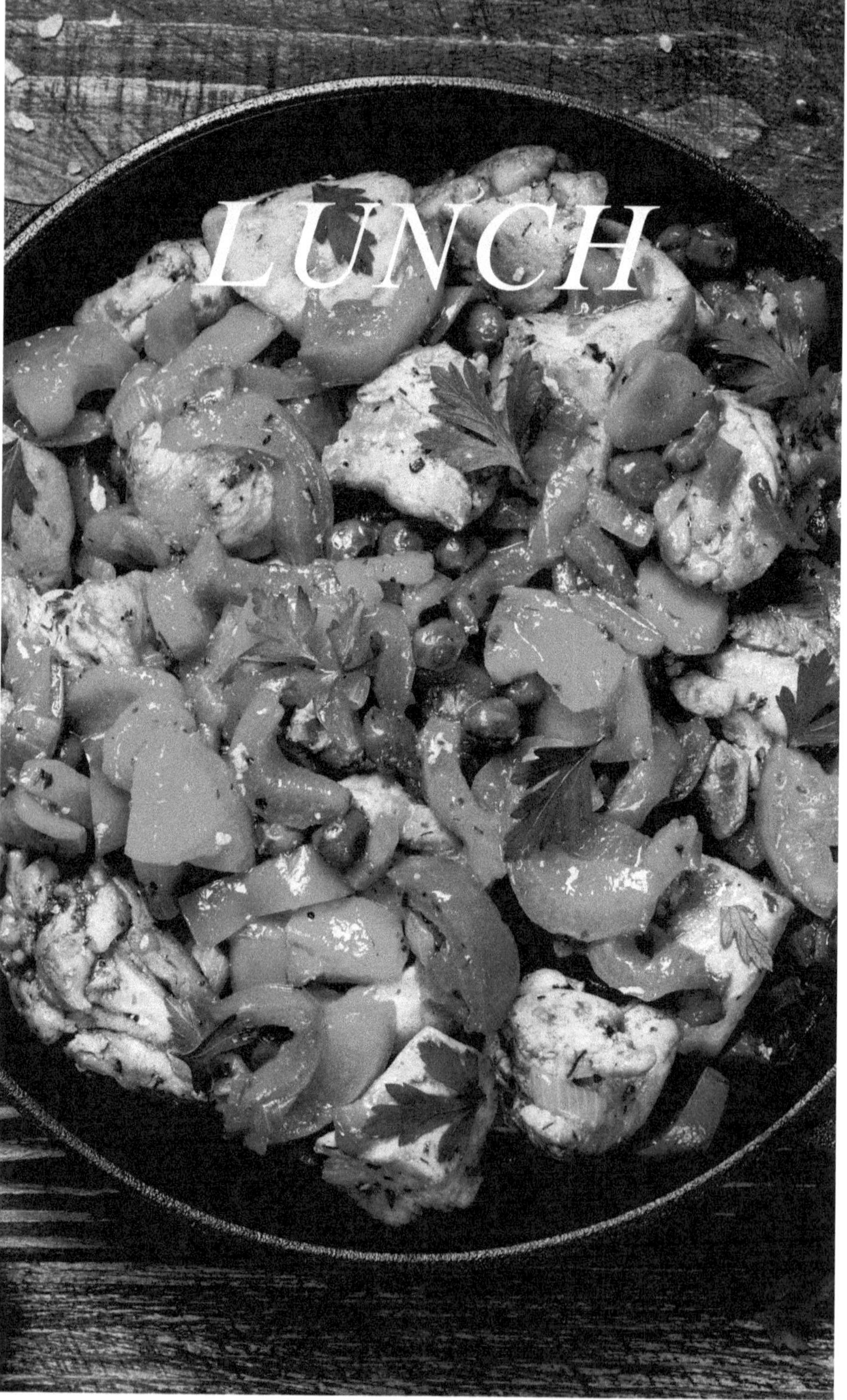
LUNCH

SMOKED MACKEREL AND LEEKS WITH HORSERADISH

INGREDIENTS

250g young potatoes, peeled and halved
2 tablespoons oil
2 big thinly sliced leeks
100g smoked mackerel with peppers, skin removed
4 eggs
Optional: 2 tbsp creamed horseradish

STEP 1 of the Method
Place the potatoes in a microwaveable bowl with a splash of water, cover, and cook for 5 minutes on high until cooked (or steam or simmer).

STEP 2 In the meantime, heat the oil in a frying pan over medium heat, add the leeks, season with salt, and simmer for 10 minutes, stirring occasionally, until softened. Add the potatoes, increase the heat, and fry for a couple of minutes to crisp them up. Break apart the mackerel.

STEP 3 Make four indentations in the leek mixture in the pan, crack an egg into each, season, and cook for 6–8 minutes, or until the whites have set and the yolks are runny. With the pan in the center of the table, serve the horseradish on the side.

SANDWICH WITH BEETROOT, HUMMUS, AND CRUNCHY CHICKPEAS

INGREDIENTS

300g pack cooked beetroot in water, drained and half sliced
400g drained chickpeas
3 tablespoons vegan pesto olive oil
a splash of vinegar (preferably white wine vinegar)
two big ciabatta breads, cut in half
2 huge handfuls salad of mixed rocket, watercress, and spinach

STEP 1 of the Method
In a food processor, combine the whole beetroot,
34 chickpeas,
2 tablespoons pesto, and 1 tablespoon oil with little seasoning to make a thick, creamy hummus.
Heat the ciabatta according to the package directions.

STEP 2 Fry the remaining chickpeas till crisp in a little oil, then set aside. Toss the salad greens in the remaining pesto and vinegar. Combine the fried chickpeas, hummus, beetroot slices, and lettuce leaves to assemble the sandwiches.

PASTA WITH PESTO AND KALE

INGREDIENTS

1 tablespoon rapeseed oil 2 finely sliced red onions
300g kale
300g wholemeal pasta (penne or mafalda are good choices)
4 tbsp soft reduced-fat cheese
4 tbsp pesto, fresh or jarred, or vegetarian substitute

STEP 1 of the Method
In a large saucepan over medium heat, heat the oil. Cook the onions for 10 minutes, or until softened and starting to caramelize. Cook for 5 minutes more, or until the kale has wilted, after adding the kale and 100 ml water.

STEP 2 Cook the pasta according to the package directions. Drain, reserving a tiny bit of the water used for cooking. Toss the pasta with the onion mixture, soft cheese, and pesto, adding a splash of the reserved cooking water if necessary to loosen it up. Season.

CACIO E PEPE GNOCCHI

INGREDIENTS

Gnocchi gnocchi 300g
2 tbsp unsalted butter
60g finely grated parmesan or vegetarian alternative
2 tsp black pepper
salad leaves (optional)

METHOD

STEP 1

In a big pot of lightly salted, boiling water, cook the gnocchi. 200ml of the cooking water should be drained and saved.

STEP 2 Melt the butter in a big skillet. Add the gnocchi, cheese, and pepper, as well as 150ml of the cooking water, and swirl rapidly until the cheese melts and the gnocchi is well coated. If you like it saucier, add more of the conserved water. Season with salt to taste. Serve the gnocchi in dishes with a mixed salad, if desired.

CHEESE AND CHILI MELTS

INGREDIENT

250g strong cheddar, grated 4 tomatoes,

roughly chopped 1 green or red chile,

deseeded and coarsely chopped 12 large

bunch coriander, leaves roughly chopped

STEP 1 of the Method
Mix the cheese, tomatoes, chili, and coriander leaves in a bowl with some spice.

STEP 2 Microwave the tortillas according to package directions to make them more malleable. Spread the cheese mixture on one half of each tortilla. Fold the other side over to form eight half-moons, then press down to seal.

VEGGIE-PACKED BAKED POTATOES

INGREDIENTS

Four medium-sized russet potatoes

Tbsp of olive oil, separated

One pinch of kosher salt

One freshly ground pinch of black pepper

two cups of baby spinach

½ piece of thinly sliced yellow bell pepper

¼ cup of feta cheese in crumbles

2 tablespoons sliced sun-dried tomatoes

Half a cup of walnut halves

3-tablespoons balsamic vinegar

One thinly sliced scallion for garnish

GUIDELINES

1.

Scrub potatoes well and pierce each one all over with a fork. Put potatoes on a plate that is safe to use in the microwave, and cook for six minutes on high. After flipping potatoes, microwave them for a further six minutes. They are ready if a knife easily inserts into the middle of each potato. If not, keep heating the potato in the microwave for two minutes at a time until the middle is cooked.

2.

Halve each potato, but do not cut off the ends. Sprinkle it with salt and pepper and drizzle with a tablespoon of olive oil. Spoon evenly over potatoes; add pepper slices, feta cheese, sun-dried tomatoes, and walnut halves.

3.

Pour the leftover olive oil and balsamic vinegar over each potato. Before serving, add a little scallions on top.

RICE & CAJUN RED BEANS

Spicy andouille sausage and beans are combined with white rice in a classic Cajun dish known as red beans and rice. For more fiber and less saturated fat, try this variation using brown rice and andouille-style chicken sausage. This recipe is a tasty way to use less meat, save money on groceries, and increase your intake of legumes without giving up meat entirely. The beans will also give you a huge surge of fiber that is good for your intestines!

INGREDIENTS
Two tablespoons pure olive oil
One chopped yellow onion
One rib celery, cut (if desired)

Three sliced links of Andouille chicken sausage
One 15.5-oz can of washed and drained tiny red beans
One teaspoon of cajun spice blend
Two cups of cooked rice ideally brown
As a garnish, fresh parsley is optional.

INSTRUCTIONS

1 Add the olive oil, onion, and celery (if using) to a nonstick skillet set over high heat. Cook for about 7 minutes, stirring often, or until onions are transparent

2.

Add the beans, sausage, cajun seasoning, and one cup of water. After giving the beans a good stir, simmer for a further seven minutes, or until they are tender. If preferred, top with parsley and serve over rice.

Lunch that's High-Fiber, Gluten-Free, and Easy to Make

SIMPLE BROCCOLI AND CHICKEN CASSEROLE

It's a fact that casseroles aren't typically considered healthful. More comforting than healthy food, casseroles are typically made with ultra-processed condensed soups (hey, sodium bomb!) and refined grains. But instead of adding extra fat, this version makes use of lean chicken tenders, broccoli, and nonfat Greek yogurt, which gives it its distinctive tang and creamy texture.

INGREDIENTS
One tablespoon pure olive oil
One pound of chicken tenders, sliced into small pieces
1/2 cup quick-cooking rice (brown preferred)
Three-quarters cup low-sodium chicken broth; one-quarter cup plain, fat-free Greek yogurt
One-third teaspoon kosher salt
One head of finely chopped broccoli
One cup of optionally shredded sharp cheddar cheese

INSTRUCTIONS

1 Heat a sizable nonstick skillet to a high temperature. Add the chicken pieces to the olive oil and heat, stirring periodically, for about two minutes, or until the chicken is browned.

2.

Stir together the rice and broth. After covering and cooking the rice for a further ten minutes on high heat, it should be soft.

3.

Add yogurt, salt, and broccoli on top. For three to four minutes, or until the broccoli is brilliant green and tender, cover and cook. dairy products Lunch that's Quick & Easy, Heart-Healthy, Gluten-Free, High-Protein, and Family Friendly

SALMON AND ASPARAGUS TACOS ON A SHEET PAN

These tasty tacos are as easy to prepare as a sheet pan meal and come together quickly. In addition, the USDA says that the asparagus provides fiber, vitamin C, and folate, and the salmon provides a healthy dosage of omega-3 fats. Actually, this gourmet dish is so easy to make that it will quickly become your lunch favorite!

INGREDIENTS
One bunch of fresh asparagus,
well cleaned, dried, and with the
tough ends cut off
Two tablespoons pure olive oil
One pinch of kosher salt
One freshly ground pinch of
black pepper
One pound of fresh salmon
Two teaspoons of low-sodium
taco seasoning

Eight of your preferred taco-sized tortillas, ideally whole-grain ones
two cups of baby spinach
Please sample your preferred green spicy sauce (optional, but highly recommended)
½ cup Greek yogurt, plain, without fat
½ thinly sliced white onion (optional)

INSTRUCTIONS

1 Start the oven at 400 degrees Fahrenheit. Use silicone mats or parchment paper to line a baking sheet.

2.

Drizzle with olive oil and place asparagus on the prepared baking sheet. Toss gently to coat evenly, then add salt and pepper for seasoning. On one side of the baking sheet, arrange the asparagus.

3.
Transfer the salmon to the opposite side of the baking sheet and evenly distribute the taco seasoning over it.

Bake for 12 to 15 minutes, or until the asparagus is crisp-tender and the salmon flakes readily.

Take it out of the oven and let it cool a bit. Gently flake the fish into generous portions using a fork.

4
One by one, reheat each tortilla for about a minute on each side in a medium skillet set over medium-high heat.

5.
To make the tacos, take a clean tortilla and arrange it on top of ¼ cup spinach, 2 to 3 asparagus

stalks, salmon, yogurt, onion, and spicy sauce (if needed). Warm up and serve.

VEGETABLE-PACKED FRITTATA

Do you have any leftover vegetables? Toss them into a frittata for an easy and wholesome weekday meal. According to the USDA, this recipe calls for broccoli, which is high in fiber and vitamin C, but you may use any vegetable you have on hand instead. According to the USDA, eggs provide a cost-effective source of protein and bind the vegetables together.

INGREDIENTS

ten huge eggs
Half a cup of skim milk
1/2 tsp kosher salt and 1/2 tsp pepper
One tablespoon pure olive oil
One broccoli head, divided into florets
two minced garlic cloves
One sliced red bell pepper
Half a cup of cherry tomatoes
One cup of baby spinach
1 tsp coarsely chopped fresh rosemary

INSTRUCTIONS

1.

Set oven temperature to 350°Fahrenheit. In a large mixing bowl, combine the eggs, milk, salt, and pepper and whisk to combine. Put aside.

2 Combine the red pepper, broccoli, garlic, and olive oil in an ovenproof nonstick skillet. Cook for about 5 minutes, stirring often, or until the broccoli is crisp-tender.

3.

Add the tomatoes, spinach, and rosemary. Cook for an additional two minutes, or until the spinach has wilted. After adding the egg mixture, bake for 10 to 15 minutes, or until the eggs are thoroughly cooked. Serve cold or warm(as desired).

HIGH-PROTEIN MACARONI AND CHEESE

Mac & cheese is a beloved food by both young and old due to its creamy and cheesy flavor, but it is also well-known for having a high fat, salt, and simple carbohydrate content. According to the Cleveland Clinic, a traditional mac and cheese may not satisfy your hunger until your next meal if it has insufficient protein. You can easily make a high-protein, gluten-free mac and cheese by replacing the white pasta with chickpea pasta and blending cottage cheese.

INGREDIENTS
One pound of whole-wheat macaroni with chickpea elbows
one cup cottage cheese (low-fat)
Two cups of cheddar cheese, shredded
Two glasses of milk, low-fat (1 percent)
Two tablespoons cornstarch
One teaspoon of kosher salt
One-half teaspoon of garlic powder

INSTRUCTIONS

Over high heat, bring a saucepan of water to a boil. When the pasta is al dente, add the macaroni and simmer, stirring regularly.

In a blender, combine the other ingredients and process for one minute, or until smooth.

After draining, put it back in the pot over medium heat.

Add the cheese sauce and stir often for two to three minutes, or until the sauce thickens. Serve right away.

ROASTED LEMON CHICKEN THIGHS WITH VEGETABLES ON A ONE-PAN

Roasting everything on one sheet pan is one of the easiest ways to get supper on the table quickly. The USDA states that chicken thighs have a bit more fat than white meat, which gives them a negative reputation. However, unlike breasts, chicken thighs have built-in portion control because they don't get too big.

INGREDIENTS

¾ teaspoon paprika

One-half teaspoon of garlic powder

One-half teaspoon of onion powder

Add extra kosher salt (¼ teaspoon) for seasoning.

¼ teaspoon of freshly ground pepper, with additional for flavoring

One tablespoon pure olive oil

Six boneless chicken thighs with no additional salt solution

Four quarts (2 cups) of grape tomatoes

Two bunches of raw asparagus with rough ends cut off

One juiced and one cut into wedges of fresh lemons

One tablespoon of freshly chopped fresh herbs (such oregano, thyme, and rosemary)

INSTRUCTIONS

1.

Set oven temperature to 425°Fahrenheit. Combine the paprika, onion, garlic, and powdered salt and pepper in a small bowl.

2.

Grease a baking sheet with a thin layer of olive oil and cover it with parchment or aluminum foil. Place sideways (the chicken thighs). Distribute the spice mixture equally on each thigh's two sides.

3.

On the opposite side of the baking sheet, place the tomatoes. Lightly sprinkle with olive oil, stirring to coat.

If necessary, evenly distribute the contents onto a single layer using a second baking sheet. Sprinkle half of the lemon juice over the whole pan and season with salt and pepper. For ten minutes, bake.

4
Take the baking sheet out of
the oven and place the
asparagus next to the
tomatoes.

Toss veggies with the leftover
lemon juice, then top chicken
with fresh herbs. Put the
asparagus back in the oven
and continue roasting it for 8
to 12 minutes, or until it
turns brilliant green and
starts to brown.

5 Present right away with
wedges of lemon.

HUNGARIAN GOULASH RECIPE

INGREDIENT

Two tablespoons pure olive oil

One chopped yellow onion

two chopped carrots

One pound of 93% lean ground turkey and one 28-oz container of diced tomatoes

A pair of dry elbow macaroni, ideally made with whole wheat

1/2 tsp paprika smoked

1/2 tsp kosher salt and 1/2 tsp freshly ground pepper

Italian parsley, optional garnish

INSTRUCTIONS

1 Heat a sizable nonstick skillet to a high temperature.

Add the olive oil, onion, and carrots. Cook, stirring regularly, for three to five minutes, or until the veggies start to soften.

2.

After adding the turkey, cook it for about 4 minutes while stirring often. Bring to a boil after adding the macaroni, tomatoes, and two cups of water.

Cook for 8 to 10 minutes, stirring now and again, or until the macaroni is al dente.

3
Add paprika, salt, and pepper for seasoning, and if you like, top with parsley.

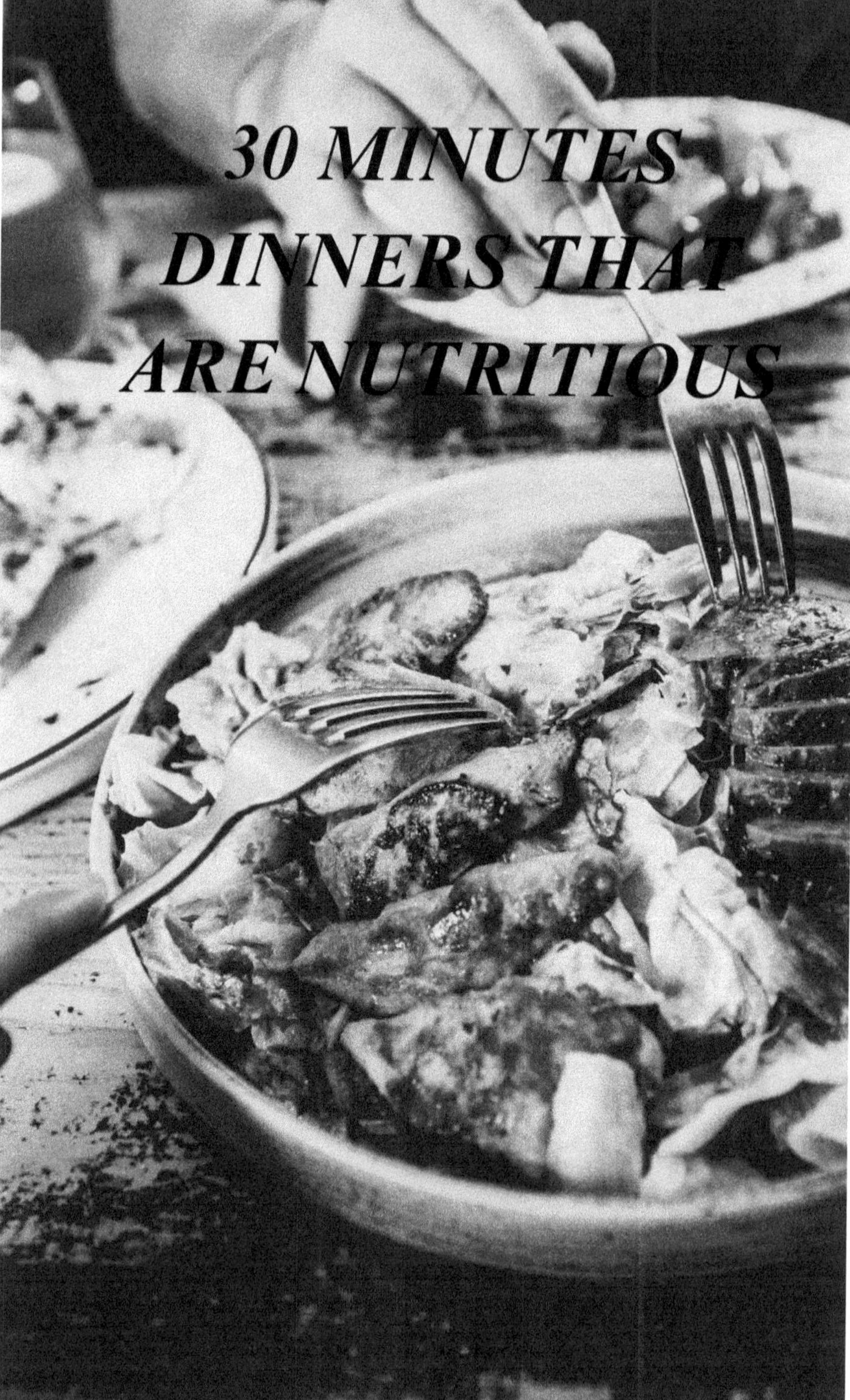
30 MINUTES
DINNERS THAT
ARE NUTRITIOUS

RIGATONI WITH VODKA

INGREDIENTS

Extra virgin olive oil (50ml)
1/4 bunch basil, plucked leaves
1 finely sliced tiny white onion
2 (500ml) cups passata
50 grams unsalted butter
2 finely sliced red chilies
1/4 cup (60ml) vodka
350ml cream thickened
500g dried rigatoni
200g grated Reggiano Parmigiano

METHOD

1.In a medium saucepan over medium heat, heat half the oil to prepare the napoletana sauce. Cook for 6-8 minutes, or until the basil and half of the onion are softened.

2.Pour in the passata after washing the bottle with 1/2 cup (125ml) water. Reduce the heat to medium-low and stew for 25-30 minutes, or until the sauce has thickened. Place aside.

3.In a separate medium saucepan over medium-low heat, combine the remaining butter, oil, chili, and onion. Cook for six to eight minutes, or until the vegetables are softened.

Pour in the vodka, it will ignite, so be careful! Remove the napoletana sauce from the heat, then add the cream and allow it to bubble and decrease for 5-7 minutes, until it is a brilliant orange color.

4.In the meantime, boil the rigatoni according to package directions until al dente.

5.After straining, add the pasta to the sauce and toss.

Toss to combine and allow to froth together before adding the parmigiano and tossing again. Serve right away.

HEALTHY FISH CURRY WITH TUMERIC AND COCONUTS

Whiting is a delicate fish that requires little cooking and complements the lightly spiced tastes of this simple recipe.

INGREDIENTS

4 chopped garlic cloves

4 sliced tiny green chilies

1 tablespoon finely minced ginger

2 tsp fresh turmeric, coarsely chopped

2 tablespoons sunflower oil

1 finely chopped onion

2 teaspoons ground coriander

2 teaspoon turmeric powder

1 teaspoon cumin

14 teaspoon ground cloves

6 green cardamom pods, 12 curry leaves (cracked), plus extra deep-fried leaves to serve

2 teaspoon turmeric powder

1 teaspoon cumin

14 teaspoon ground cloves

400ml coconut milk can
1 cup fish stock (250ml)
600g sand whiting filets or skin-on whiting filets, cut into 4 cm pieces
One lime juice

To serve, steamed basmati rice
To serve, coriander leaves

METHOD
1.Pulverize the garlic, chili, ginger, and turmeric in a mortar and pestle.

2.In a deep frypan over medium heat, heat the oil. Cook, stirring constantly, for 3-4 minutes, or until the onion is softened.

Cook, stirring constantly, for 3-4 minutes, or until the chili paste is aromatic.

Cook, stirring constantly, for another 2 minutes after adding the spices and curry leaves.

Bring the coconut milk and stock to a simmer.
3.Simmer for ten minutes, stirring now and again, until somewhat reduced.Cook for 4 minutes, or until the fish is just done.

Remove the pan from the burner or heat. Season with lime juice and salt to taste.
4.Serve with rice and garnish with coriander and deep-fried curry leaves.

SAINT PETER'S FISH SOUP

This fish soup is the perfect winter warmer.

INGREDIENTS

1 small entire triggerfish, red mullet, red gurnard, blue spot flathead, or bream, cleaned and scaled

1 red spot whiting, cleaned and scaled

Extra virgin olive oil, 120ml

1 tiny crab (blue swimmer, brown, or sand)

10 king prawn shells and heads

1 thinly sliced onion

3 smashed garlic cloves

1 neatly sliced tiny fennel bulb

2 tablespoons tomato paste

2 roughly chopped tomatoes

a quarter bunch thyme sprigs

5 sprigs lemon thyme (optional)

1 teaspoon roasted fennel seeds

anise with two stars
4 dried ground bush tomato (optionally replace with smoked paprika)
Saffron strands, pinched
To taste, lemon juice

ROUILLE
1 roasted and peeled red capsicum
1 long red chili (seeded)
2 peeled and chopped potatoes
50g macadamia nuts, toasted
5 cloves garlic
Optional: 2 dried ground bush tomatoes
14 teaspoon smoked paprika
Saffron threads, pinch
Extra virgin olive oil (210ml)
To taste, lemon juice

GARNISHES FOR FINISHING

500g small waxy potatoes, such as Dutch cream or bintje, skinned
on 5 x 120g cleaned and scaled red mullet

200g roe of John Dory
400g cleaned cuttlefish or squid tentacles
500g de-sanded (purged) pipis or clams
10 peeled and deveined king prawns
50g ghee
250g best available fish liver (for example, John Dory, grouper, or cod)

TO BE SERVED
1 loaf of high-quality
rye bread
100g cold salted
cultured butter of high
quality
250g salad greens with
mixed herbs

METHOD
1.To make the soup
base, slice the fish into
small pieces using a
sharp cleaver.

2.Heat 100ml olive oil in
a big, wide, heavy-
based pot and cook the
crab and prawn shells
and heads for 10-12
minutes, or until
browned. Set aside in a
mixing dish.

3.Return the saucepan
to medium heat and
add the chopped fish
in the same oil. Cook
for 10 minutes, or
until browned all over,
seasoning liberally
with salt. Set aside
alongside the
shellfish.

Cook for 5 minutes, or
until the tomato paste
is aromatic. Cover with
water and add all of
the fish and shellfish,
as well as the
additional ingredients
(excluding the lemon
juice).

Bring to a boil, covered
with a lid. When it
reaches a boil, cover
and simmer for 20
minutes over high
heat.

5.After pulsing the stock in a food processor or straining it through a mouli, taste and add salt, lemon juice, and pepper as needed.

GODDESS BOWLS

INGREDIENTS

1/2 pound asparagus, trimmed

2 tablespoons extra-virgin olive oil, split

ground black pepper, freshly ground

1 pound skinless boneless chicken breasts

1 teaspoon garlic powder

1 teaspoon dried oregano

TO BE DRESSED

1 cup of mayonnaise

1 cup of Greek yogurt

1 1/2 cups chopped basil

1/2 cup parsley, chopped

1/4 cup chopped chives (plus additional for garnish)

1 cup lemon juice

2 garlic cloves, finely chopped

FOR THE BOWLS

4 cup brown rice, cooked

1 sliced avocado 1 cup halved cherry tomatoes

DIRECTIONS

Preheat the oven to 425°F for the first step, roasting the asparagus. Toss asparagus with 1 tablespoon oil and season with salt and pepper on a large baking sheet. Bake for 15 minutes, or until the asparagus is tender.

Step 2 Cook the chicken: In a large skillet over medium heat, heat the remaining olive oil. Season the chicken on both sides with garlic powder, dried oregano, salt, and pepper. Cook until brown and cooked through, about 8 minutes per side, in a heated skillet. Remove from the heat and let aside for 10 minutes before cutting into strips.

Step 3 To make the dressing, combine mayonnaise, yogurt, basil, parsley, chives, lemon juice, and garlic in a food processor. Season with salt and pepper to taste after pulsing until smooth.

Step 4: Assemble the bowls: Divide the rice among four serving bowls. Avocado, cherry tomatoes, grilled chicken, and roasted asparagus go on top. Pour dressing over each bowl. Serve right away.

EVERYTHING BAGEL CRUSTED SALMON

INGREDIENTS

4 skin-on salmon filets (6 oz.)
Kosher salt is kosher salt.
ground black pepper, freshly ground
2 tablespoons spicy harissa paste
3 heaping tablespoons everything bagel seasoning
3 tbsp. Extra virgin olive oil, 1 1/2 oz. softened cream cheese (approximately 3 tbsp.), 1 small onion, roughly chopped,

1/4 cup coarsely chopped fresh dill, 2 tbsp. fresh lemon juice, 2 oz. arugula
1 tiny cucumber, split into 1/4"-thick rounds 6 oz. cherry tomatoes, halved
1 tbsp. finely chopped drained capers 1 oz. thin bagel chips

DIRECTIONS

Step 1 Preheat the oven to 450°F with a rack in the center. Preheat a big cast-iron skillet on a rack.

Step 2: Pat fish dry and season with 1 teaspoon salt and a pinch of pepper all over. Spread harissa on top of the salmon flesh. Sprinkle everything bagel seasoning over each filet.

Step 3 Remove the skillet from the oven with care and drizzle with 2 tablespoons of oil. With the skin side down, place the salmon on the skillet. Bake for 10 to 12 minutes, or until the flesh is opaque and easily flakes with a fork.

Meanwhile, in a small mixing bowl, combine cream cheese, half of the shallot, 1 tablespoon dill, 1 tablespoon lemon juice, 2 tablespoons water, and the remaining 1

1 tablespoon oil; season with salt. Soak the remaining shallots in the remaining 1 tablespoon lemon juice in a separate small bowl.

Step 5 Toss arugula, tomato, cucumber, capers, marinated shallots, and remaining 3 tablespoons dill in a large mixing dish.

Toss in half of the dressing, then top with bagel chips.

Step 6 Arrange salmon on plates. Serve with the salad and the remaining dressing on the side.

BLACK BEAN TOSTADAS

INGREDIENTS

2 (15-oz.) cans rinsed and drained black beans

8 tortillas

2 cups shredded pepper jack cheese

sliced avocado

Spicy sauce

DIRECTIONS

Step 1

Preheat the oven to 350 degrees Fahrenheit. Add the beans and 1 cup of water to a small saucepan set over medium heat. Bring to a simmer and cook for 10 minutes, or until the beans are thoroughly warmed. Smash with a wooden spoon until most of the beans are smashed but some are still intact. To achieve

a smoother consistency, add more water as needed.

Step 2 In the meantime, arrange tostadas on a large baking sheet and evenly sprinkle with cheese. Bake for 5 minutes, or until the cheese is melted.

Step 3

Tostadas should be topped with beans, avocado slices, and hot sauce.

TACOS WITH CRISPY CHIPOTLE CHICKEN

Putting cheese right in your skillet may seem counterintuitive, but it works! Once removed from the heat, the cheese begins to firm and crisp up, resulting in the texture of a crunchy taco shell that is also extremely cheesy. After these, you'll be making tacos every night of the week.

INGREDIENTS

RANCH AVOCADO SAUCE
a single avocado
1 seeded and chopped jalapeno
2 garlic cloves
1/2 cup fresh cilantro, packed
1 cup buttermilk
1 cup sour cream
One lime juice
Kosher salt
ground black pepper, freshly ground

TACOS
1 tablespoon of extra-virgin olive oil
1 medium sliced yellow onion
3 minced garlic cloves
1 pound ground chicken

1 chopped chipotle chile in adobo sauce, plus 2 tbsp adobo sauce

1 teaspoon chili powder

1 teaspoon cumin
Kosher salt is kosher salt.
ground black pepper, freshly ground
8 small corn tortillas, 3 cup shredded cheddar
To serve, fresh cilantro leaves

DIRECTIONS
RANCH AVOCADO SAUCE
Step 1 Puree avocado, jalapeno, garlic, cilantro, buttermilk, sour cream, and lime

juice in a food processor or blender until smooth; season with salt and pepper.

Step 2 Place the sauce in an airtight container. Store in the fridge until you're ready to use it.
Step 3: Make Ahead: Sauce can be made up to 3 days ahead of time. Store in the refrigerator.

TACOS
Step 1 In a big skillet, heat the oil over medium heat. Cook, stirring constantly, until the onion is softened, about 5 minutes. Cook, stirring constantly, until the garlic is aromatic, about 1 minute more.
Cook, breaking up the flesh with a wooden spoon, until the chicken is no longer pink, about 8 minutes.

Season with salt and pepper and stir in the chipotle chile, adobo sauce, chili powder, and cumin. Take the pan off the burner or heat.

Step 2 Melt about 1/4 cup cheese in a small nonstick skillet over medium heat in a circle the size of your tortillas. Put a tortilla over the top. Spread roughly 2 tablespoons cheese on one half of the tortilla and some chicken stuffing on the other. Cook until the bottom

cheese begins to crisp, about 4 minutes. Press to keep the taco closed after folding the cheese-covered half up and over the chicken.

Cook for 1 minute until warmed through, then flip and cook for 1 minute more until the second side is warmed through. Place on a platter. Rep with the remaining tacos.

Step 3: Garnish tacos with cilantro. Accompany with avocado ranch sauce.

QUESADILLAS WITH BLACK BEANS

Are you in a hurry? These filling quesadillas are ready in 15 minutes. We prefer them with black beans, but pinto beans also work well. If you like things spicy, use pepper Jack cheese in the filling. Serve with a dollop of sour cream and a salad of mixed greens.

INGREDIENTS

1 rinsed 15-ounce can black beans

12 cup shredded Monterey Jack cheese (preferred)

1/2 cup freshly prepared salsa (see Tip), split

4 whole-wheat tortillas, 8 in.

divided 2 teaspoons canola oil

1 chopped ripe avocado

DIRECTIONS

In a medium mixing dish, combine the beans, cheese, and 1/4 cup salsa.

Lay out the tortillas on a surface for work. There should be 1/2 cup of filling on half of each tortilla. Tortillas should be gently folded in half.

Heat one teaspoon of oil in a big, nonstick skillet over medium heat. Cook, flipping once, until golden on both sides, about 2 to 4 minutes total.

To keep warm, transfer to a cutting board and tent with foil.

Repeat with the rest of the oil and quesadillas. Serve the quesadillas with thc leftover salsa and avocado.

CHICKEN ENCHILADA-STUFFED SPAGHETTI SQUASH

INGREDIENTS

2 boneless, skinless chicken breasts (8 oz.)

1 spaghetti squash, halved lengthwise and seeded, 2 1/2 to 3 pounds

14 cup red enchilada sauce (divided)

1 medium diced zucchini

1 cup pepper Jack cheese, shredded

This 5-ingredient spaghetti squash recipe is a filling low-carb substitute for taco night. Skip.

Step 2 and add 2 1/2 cups cooked chicken into the filling if you have leftover prepared chicken. Search for enchilada sauce, like

Hatch brand, that has less than 300 mg of salt per serving.

Preheat the oven to $450°F$ and place racks in the upper and bottom thirds of the oven.

In a medium saucepan, cover the chicken with water and bring to a boil. Cover, lower heat to low, and gently simmer for 10 to 15 minutes, or until an instant-read thermometer inserted into the thickest part registers 165 degrees F.

GNOCCHI CAULIFLOWER OREGANATA SHRIMP

On busy nights, this cauliflower gnocchi meal is ready in minutes. The soft pasta is paired with sautéed shrimp in a flavor-packed sauce. If you don't like shrimp, substitute rotisserie chicken.

INGREDIENTS

1 (12 oz.) bag frozen cauliflower gnocchi

1 pint halved grape tomatoes

1 tablespoon extra virgin olive oil

2 tablespoons garlic mince

14 teaspoon dried oregano

1 teaspoon salt

1 pound cooked peeled shrimp (about 31-40 per pound; thawed if frozen)

DIRECTIONS

Gnocchi should be cooked according to package specifications.

In a large microwave-safe bowl,

combine the tomatoes, oil, garlic, oregano, and salt. Microwave on High for 1 minute, or until softened. Incorporate the gnocchi and shrimp.

STUFFED SWEET POTATOES WITH CHICKEN CURRY

To make these simple loaded baked potatoes, use convenience ingredients like cooked chicken (either leftover or purchased) and store-bought curry sauce. This recipe calls for cauliflower, but feel free to use any vegetables you have on hand for a quick and easy dinner. You can also substitute russets for the sweet potatoes.

INGREDIENTS

4 medium sweet potatoes (about 8 ounces each)

12 cup curry sauce from Madras

12 cup cooked cauliflower, diced

8 ounces warmed chopped cooked chicken

4 teaspoons fresh cilantro, chopped

DIRECTIONS

With a fork, pierce the potatoes all over. Microwave on Medium for 20 minutes, stirring once or twice. (Alternatively, bake potatoes until soft, 45 minutes to 1 hour at 425°F.) Allow to cool somewhat on a clean cutting board.

To open the potato, make a lengthwise cut with a kitchen towel to protect your hands, but don't cut all the way through. Pinch the ends together to expose the flesh.

Each potato should be topped with curry sauce, cauliflower, chicken, and cilantro. Serve hot.

MUSHROOMS & CREAMY CHICKEN

Whether you have wild mushrooms from the farmers' market, cultivated maitake or shiitake mushrooms from the supermarket, or simply some baby bellas on hand, this healthful creamy chicken recipe is excellent with any of them. Over mashed potatoes or whole-wheat egg noodles are served.

Are Mushrooms Healthy?

While mushrooms may not fit into the "eat the rainbow" campaign, these earthy fungi have numerous health benefits. Mushrooms are high in B vitamins and have been proved to reduce inflammation and improve gut health.

INGREDIENTS

4 4- to 5-ounce chicken cutlets (see Tips)

4 cups mushroom mixture, sliced if large

12 cup white wine, dry

12 c. thick cream

2 tbsp fresh parsley, freshly chopped

DIRECTIONS

Season the chicken with 1/4 teaspoon kosher salt and 1/4 teaspoon black pepper. In a large skillet over medium heat.

heat 1 tablespoon canola oil. Cook the chicken, rotating once, for 7 to 10 minutes, or until browned and cooked through. Place on a platter.

Cook, stirring regularly, until the liquid has evaporated, about 4 minutes, with 1 tablespoon oil and mushrooms in the pan.

Turn the heat up to high, pour in the wine, and simmer until the wine has evaporated, about 4 minutes.

Reduce the heat to medium and mix in the cream, any accumulated chicken juice, and 1/4 teaspoon salt and pepper.

Return the chicken to the pan and toss it around to coat with the sauce. Serve the chicken with the sauce on top and dusted with parsley.

Make your own chicken cutlets using two 8- to 10-ounce boneless, skinless chicken breasts. Save the tenders (the strip of meat on the bottom of the breast) for another occasion.

Each breast should be cut in half crosswise. Place between two plastic wrap layers.

Pound the beef with a meat mallet or a skillet until it's about 1/2 inch thick.

SUMMER SQUASH, FETA, AND BASIL GRILLED PIZZA

Spreading roasted red pepper hummus on this simple grilled pizza provides a quick and easy base for soft summer squash and salty feta bits. The best part? This nutritious pizza takes about 20 minutes to prepare.

INGREDIENTS

1 pound whole-wheat pizza dough

12 cup hummus with roasted red peppers

2 cups summer squash, thinly sliced

up feta cheese, crumbled

12 cup fresh basil, sliced

Garnish with ground pepper

DIRECTIONS

Preheat the grill to medium-high temperature.

On a lightly floured board, roll the dough into a 12-inch oval.

Place on a large baking sheet that has been lightly floured. To the grill, add the dough, hummus, squash, and feta.

Grease the grill rack. Place the crust on the grill. Close the lid and simmer for 1 to 2 minutes, or until puffed and gently browned.

Turn the crust over with tongs. Spread the hummus on the crust and top with the squash and feta.

Cook for 2 to 3 minutes more, or until the cheese is melted and the crust is lightly browned on the bottom.

Place the pizza back on the baking sheet. If desired, garnish with basil and pepper.

TURKEY TWIST PIE

INGREDIENTS
500g chargrilled veggies, chopped, frozen

130g box roast turkey slices 250g tub ricotta

7 sheets filo pastry (270g)

METHOD
STEP 1
Preheat the oven to 200C/180C fan/gas 6.

Fry the vegetables in 1 tablespoon of olive oil for eight to Ten minutes. Chop the turkey and combine it with the vegetables and ricotta, seasoning well.

Oil a work surface and overlap four filo sheets to make a rectangle 40 x 60cm.

Brush the remaining sheets with oil and place them on top.

Filling should be spooned down the bottom third, folded in the short sides, rolled up, and twisted into a spiral.

Brush with extra oil and bake for 45 minutes on a nonstick baking sheet.

FRITTATA WITH GOAT CHEESE, PEAS, AND BEANS

This recipe is ideal for a quick supper because you're likely to have all of the ingredients on hand.

INGREDIENTS

300g frozen peas and beans mixture

8 large eggs, plus a dash of milk

100g log goat's cheese, rind included, or feta

1-2 tbsp chopped mint a drizzle of oil

METHOD

STEP 1
Preheat the grill to medium heat. Cook for 4 minutes, or until the peas and beans are just cooked, then drain well.

Combine the eggs, a splash of milk, and spices in a mixing bowl. Slice 4 thin, round slices of goat's cheese (approximately half the log), roughly chop or crumble the remaining into bits, and stir into the eggs with the vegetables and herbs.

STEP 2 Preheat an oven proof shallow pan with a light coating of oil. Pour in the egg mixture and simmer for 8-10 minutes,or until there is just a little un-set mix on the surface.

Place the slices of goat's cheese on top, then grill until firm, golden, and the cheese is bubbling.

RECIPE SUGGESTIONS

PASTA WITH GOAT'S CHEESE AND GREENS
Boil 400g pasta for 4 minutes, then add the bean mixture. While draining, leave some of the cooking water.

Meanwhile, in 3 tbsp oil, sauté 2 sliced garlic cloves and 1-2 finely chopped red chilies.

Return the pasta to the pan, toss in the garlic, chili, and oil, and add a splash of water to loosen. Stir in the goat's cheese, all of it chopped this time. Allow it to melt for 1 minute before stirring in a handful of rockets.

Serve with a drizzle of extra virgin olive oil and adjust the seasoning to suit.

LASAGNA LENTIL VEGETARIAN

This vegetarian lentil lasagne is the most straightforward lasagna you'll ever cook. Make it on a weeknight with ready-made soup, pesto, and canned lentils! There is no pre-cooking at all. Simply layer it and bake.

Making the Easiest Lentil Lasagne Ever
So there you have it. This lasagne is made with some convenience ingredients, but not the usual jarred bechamel/bolognese mix.

Fresh tomato soup and canned or deli pesto are far more appealing and no less convenient.

And if you use ready-made lentils, pre-shredded cheese, and lasagne noodles that don't need to be cooked ahead of time, you won't have to do anything at all.
You'll simply open your packages and start layering things.

INGREDIENTS

1 package no-prep lasagne sheets

(2.5 cups) 600 mL Creamy tomato soup in a can

1 cup Lentils precooked from a can or bag

190 g (7 oz) green pesto jar

a few handfuls of cheese

GUIDELINES

Set the oven's temperature to 180 degrees Celsius, or 350 degrees F.

There is no need to pre-cook or pre-mix anything. Simply layer everything cold.

Pour some soup into the bottom of the pan, then add the first layer of pasta sheets.

My layers were as follows: tomato soup covered with lentils / pesto / REPEAT / a topping

created with the remaining tomato soup, cheese, and the last dollops of pesto

Bake for about 50 minutes with the pan covered.

Please keep in mind that this recipe is best suited for a smaller lasagna tray or perhaps a brownie pan.

If you wish to use a full-size deep lasagna pan, double the ingredients.

This is easily veganized by substituting the cheese layer with crunchy breadcrumbs or vegan parmesan and using vegan soup and pesto!

CHEESY TORTELLINI BAKE

INGREDIENTS

1 pound cheese tortellini (from the refrigerated area)

marinara sauce, 24 oz.
1 cup shredded mozzarella cheese

1/4 cup chopped flat-leaf parsley

4 oz. slices of fresh mozzarella

INSTRUCTIONS

Oven temperature: set to 350 degrees.

Set aside a 9x9 baking dish coated with cooking spray.

Cook the tortellini pasta for 3 minutes in boiling water. Rinse and drain.

Combine the cooked tortellini, marinara sauce, shredded mozzarella cheese, and parsley in a medium mixing basin.

Stir gently until the mixture is mixed.

spoon or transfer mixture into a baking dish. If you'd like, sprinkle extra parsley and fresh mozzarella slices over top.

Bake for 30 minutes, uncovered, in a preheated oven, or until the pasta is heated through and the cheeses are melted.

Serve hot!

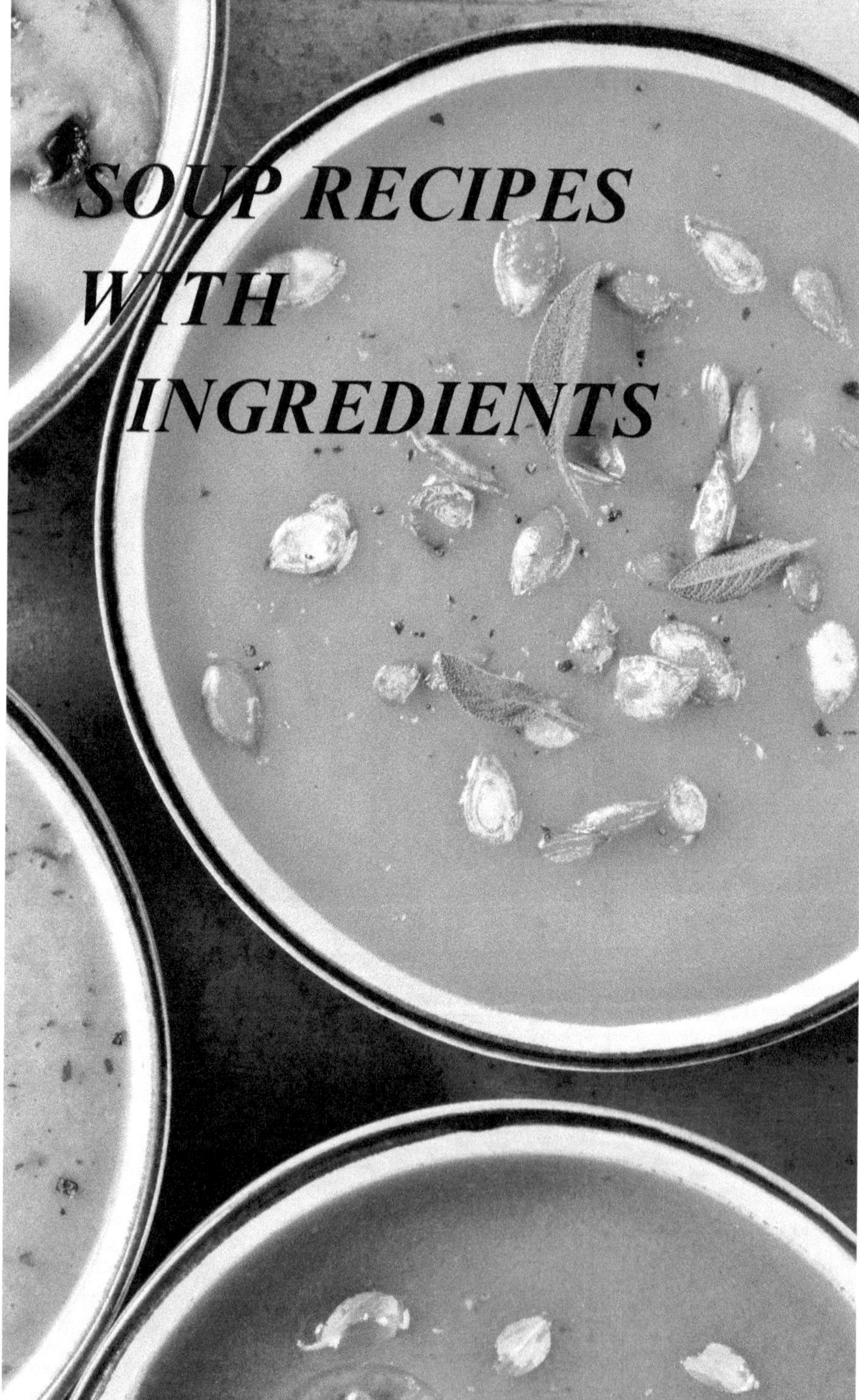
SOUP RECIPES
WITH
INGREDIENTS

WHITE CHICKEN CHILI WITH 5 INGREDIENTS

This 5-ingredient white chicken chili recipe is quick and simple to prepare, full of flavor, and always a crowd pleaser!

This dish is as simple as they get. Simply combine all of the ingredients, bring the soup to a simmer, ladle it up while it's hot, and top with your favorite toppings to serve. I've definitely prepared this dish at least a hundred times over the years, and it never fails to satisfy. If you want to save the leftovers or prepare a large quantity for fast meal prep, it also freezes and reheats wonderfully.

I swear to you, this dish is always a hit. Let's get started!

WHITE CHICKEN CHILI WITH 5 INGREDIENTS:

To create this white chicken chili dish, you'll need the following five ingredients (plus a lot of toppings):

Any form of chopped or shredded chicken will suffice. I usually shred rotisserie chicken or use frozen chicken from my Instant Pot Shredded Chicken or Baked Chicken Breasts recipes.

Salsa verde: Use homemade or store-bought salsa verde. I should mention that the heat level of store-bought versions of roasted salsa verde can vary greatly. So, if you like a milder soup, I would absolutely recommend looking for a milder salsa.

Beans: You can use any kind of beans in this chicken chili recipe.l usually use white beans (Great Northerns), but pinto, garbanzo, or black beans would also be great.

Because the ingredient list is so brief, I recommend choosing a high-quality brand of chicken or vegetable stock, whatever you prefer. Cumin: To further smooth out the ingredients in the salsa verde, we'll add a pinch of cumin to the broth.

Finally, I recommend putting a generous amount of whatever toppings you enjoy the most! I usually always top my soup with cilantro and fresh avocado.

However, crumbled tortilla chips, diced red or green onions, sour cream, shredded cheese (sharp cheddar, Monterrey Jack, or a Mexican-blend), crumbled cotija cheese, and/or sliced jalapenos are also tasty additions!

DIRECTIONS FOR MAKING THIS SOUP:

Simply combine 5 ingredients to make this 5-ingredient white chicken chili recipe...

Mix all ingredients together.In a large stockpot, combine chicken stock, shredded chicken, beans, salsa, and cumin.
Bring to a boil. Cook the soup over high heat until it reaches a simmer. Reduce the heat to medium-low and continue to cook for 5 minutes.
Serve. Then spoon the soup into serving bowls and top with your choice garnishes.

POSSIBLE VARIATIONS: There are so many different ways to customize this soup recipe! Feel free to, for example...

increase the amount of veggies to the dish.If you want to add some extra veggies to this soup,
 I recommend diced poblano peppers, onions, and/or potatoes (you can use frozen hash brown potatoes as a shortcut).

Make it in the slow cooker or the Instant Pot. This soup actually only needs to be stirred and warmed. So, if you prefer to use one of those appliances, let it simmer on low in the Crock-Pot or use the sauté option on your Instant Pot.

BLACK BEAN SOUP WITH 5 INGREDIENTS

Black bean soups are one of my favorite dishes.

Black bean soups are typically quick, healthful, and full of spices and flavor – all of which I enjoy!! Even so, the notion of a 5-ingredient black bean soup sounded appealing.

Therefore, I carried it out. Nonetheless, in 20 minutes. (Bonus!)

Can you name the five ingredients?

I had intended to prepare the soup with canned black beans (but you could use fresh if you soak them overnight), salsa, cumin, fresh cilantro, and veggie broth. But after I mixed in the first four ingredients and tasted it, I noticed that even without the veggie broth, the soup was delicious and thick and well-seasoned!

Granted, I used the entire can of beans, including the liquid, which is just water and salt and is completely safe to consume (and a great thickening for soup!). If, on the other hand, you insist on draining your beans, hakuna
 matata. Simply add one additional cup of vegetable or chicken broth.

So, since I had an additional ingredient, I added a little minced garlic, because I'm persuaded (along with Friends) that everything tastes better with a little extra garlic. ;)
But I will say that the important element in this soup is salsa that you enjoy. Add some nice hot salsa if you like spicy soup. If you prefer something milder, go for it. You can

add salsa verde if you truly like the tomatillo flavor.

I used store-bought salsa in the name of a true 20-minute supper. If you need a recommendation, I propose the national brand Herdez. Their "Casera" salsa (available in mild, medium, or hot) and my personal favorite, Chipotle, are both excellent in recipes. It's certainly the most readily available brand I've found that I enjoy, and it's also among the most economical.
Overall, this meal is a fantastic start to our 5 Ingredient Soup.

FIVE CANS SOUPS

My family adores this canned soup dish. It's perfect for football gatherings and a fresh take on chips and dip! Serve with your preferred corn chips.

INGREDIENTS

1 (15-ounce) can of premade chili with beans

1 can whole kernel corn (14 oz.)

1 can (10 3/4 oz) vegetable beef soup

1 can tomato soup (10 3/4 oz.)

1 can (10 oz.) chopped tomatoes with green chile peppers

DIRECTIONS

In a saucepan over medium-high heat, combine chili, corn, vegetable beef soup, tomato soup, and diced tomatoes with green chile peppers; simmer until heated, 5 to 10 minutes.

MENUDO

This dish is dependent on how much of each component you use. It all depends on how much money you want to make. This recipe takes some time to prepare and cook, but it is well worth the effort. The spices are always chosen based on how hot or spicy you prefer your cuisine. The following day, it tastes even better. Increase the ingredients if you want to produce more. Reduce the ingredients if you want less. I discovered this on my own, and my Mexican husband likes it. It will satisfy even the most ardent fan of Mexican cuisine.

INGREDIENTS

2 pound tripe beef

2 chopped onions

4 cans white hominy (15 oz.)

14 tsp chili powder

season with salt and pepper to taste

DIRECTIONS

Combine the tripe and onions in a 16-quart saucepan. Pour half of the water into the kettle. Cook for about 2 hours on low heat, or until the tripe is soft.

To taste, add the hominy, chili powder, and salt and pepper. Cook for another 45 minutes to an hour, covered, to allow the flavors to blend.

If desired, serve with fresh onions, corn tortillas, and lemon.

SOUP WITH ITALIAN BEEF AND BARLEY

The most delicious beef barley soup. Thickens only with barley. Slow cooker yields the greatest results. Serve with a salad and parmesan Parmesan on top.

INGREDIENTS

can (8 oz.) tomato sauce

2 pound beef chuck roast cubed

34 cup pearl barley, uncooked

5 c. water

season with salt and pepper to taste

4 beef bouillon cubes, crushed

12 onion, diced

DIRECTIONS

Combine beef, water, bouillon, onion, tomato sauce, barley, salt, and pepper in a slow cooker.

Cook on Low for 5 hours, covered.

SOUP WITH HAM AND POTATOES

A buddy gave me this ham and potato soup recipe. It's delicious and simple to prepare. What's the best part? You may add more ingredients like carrots and ham and it will still taste wonderful.
It's not only a terrific way to use up leftover cooked ham, but it's also simple to personalize with any ingredients you have on hand.

INGREDIENTS

3 cup chopped
 and peeled potatoes

3cup water

3cup cooked diced ham

1 cup celery, diced

1 cup finely diced onion
2 tbsp granules chicken bouillon
1 teaspoon black or white pepper, or to taste
1 teaspoon salt, or more to taste
5 teaspoons melted butter
5 tbsp. all-purpose flour
2 quarts milk

DIRECTIONS

In a stockpot, combine potatoes, water, ham, celery, and onion. Bring to a boil; reduce to a medium heat and cook until the potatoes are cooked, 10 to 15 minutes. Combine the chicken bouillon, pepper, and salt in a mixing bowl.

Heat a different saucepan over medium-low heat to melt the butter.
Cook for approximately a minute, stirring regularly, or until the flour thickens. Cook and whisk for 4 to 5 minutes, or until the milk is thick.

Pour the milk mixture into the stockpot and heat, stirring constantly, until warmed through.

ITALIAN-STYLE STEWED TOMATOES

INGREDIENTS

1 cup carrots, sliced

14 teaspoon of salt

14 teaspoon black pepper, ground

1 (14.5 oz) can undrained Great Northern beans

2 diced tiny zucchini

2 cups packed, washed, and torn spinach

DIRECTIONS

Over medium-high heat, heat a stock pot or Dutch oven.

Cook and stir until the sausage and garlic are browned, 5 to 7 minutes.

Season with salt and pepper and stir in the broth, tomatoes, and carrots.
After lowering
the heat to medium-low and covering, cook for fifteen minutes.

127

CHICKEN NOODLE SOUP IN MINUTES

When you don't have time to cook your soup from scratch, this chicken noodle soup recipe is a great option.

Whether you're feeling under the weather or simply in need of some consolation, nothing beats homemade chicken noodle soup for warming you up from the inside out. In less than 40 minutes, you can serve the best chicken noodle soup you've ever eaten with this easy recipe.

INGREDIENTS FOR CHICKEN NOODLE SOUP
This top-rated chicken noodle soup recipe calls for the following ingredients:

Diced onions and chopped celery are sautéed in butter until fragrant and soft in the first step of this chicken noodle soup recipe.
Broth: A combination of chicken and vegetable broths is used in this chicken noodle soup dish. You can use either one or the other if you're short on time or ingredients.

Chicken: Of course, chicken is required.For a less expensive option, you may substitute any leftover rotisserie chicken for the cooked chicken breasts.

Noodles: Do not add the noodles too early, as they will get mushy if cooked for too long.

Carrots: Carrots are added at the end of cooking to retain their crispness and add a flash of brilliant color and flavor. If you prefer your carrots tender, add them to the sautéed vegetables at the beginning.

This chicken noodle soup dish is enhanced with the warm, earthy flavor of dried basil and oregano.

Noodles That Work Best For Chicken Noodle Soup
The usual choice for chicken noodle soup is egg noodles. Rotini and fusilli would also work well, but in a pinch, use whatever you have on hand.

PERSONALIZE TO YOUR LIKING

We adore how easy this chicken noodle soup dish is. You may, however, get creative with spices and condiments. Bay leaves, garlic, herbes de Provence, rosemary, and thyme are popular additions, according to reviewers.

Utilize what you currently have, and make do. This recipe lends itself to simple, cost-effective substitutions. Replace cooked chicken breasts with rotisserie chicken, broth with water and bouillon cubes, or oil with butter.

INGREDIENTS
1 tablespoon melted butter

12 cup finely chopped onion

12 cup celery, chopped

(14.5 oz.) 4 cans chicken broth

(14.5 oz) 1 can vegetable broth

12 pound cooked chicken breast, chopped

1 pound egg noodles

1 cup carrots, sliced

12 tsp dried basil

12 tsp dried oregano

season with salt and black pepper to taste

DIRECTIONS

In a large pot over medium heat, melt the butter. Cook until the onion and celery are barely soft, about 5 minutes.

Combine the chicken broth, vegetable broth, chicken, egg noodles, carrots, basil, oregano, salt, and pepper in a mixing bowl. Bring to a boil while stirring all the time.
Simmer for 20 minutes on reduced heat.

GRATINÉE FRENCH ONION SOUP

INGREDIENTS

4 tbsp. melted butter

2 big finely sliced red onions

2 big finely sliced sweet onions

1 teaspoon sea salt

1 can (48 fluid ounces) chicken broth

1 can of beef broth (14 oz.)

12 cup of red wine

1 tsp. Worcestershire sauce

1 fresh parsley sprigs

1 fresh thyme leaf sprigs

one bay leaf

1 tbsp. balsamic vinegar

season with salt and freshly ground black pepper to taste

4 pieces thick French bread

8 slices room temperature Gruyère cheese

12 cup room temperature shredded Asiago cheese

4 paprika pinches

In a large pot over medium-high heat, melt the butter. Stir in the red and sweet onions, as well as the salt. Cook, stirring regularly, for 35 minutes, or until onions are caramelized and almost syrupy.

Combine the chicken broth, beef broth, red wine, and Worcestershire sauce in a mixing bowl.

Wrap kitchen twine around the parsley, thyme, and bay leaf and add to the saucepan. Simmer for 20 minutes, stirring occasionally, over medium heat. Take out and discard the herb bundle. Reduce the heat and season with salt and pepper.

While you prepare the toast, cover the soup and keep it heated over low heat.

Preheat the oven's broiler and position an oven rack about 6 inches from the heat source. Place bread slices on a baking pan and broil for 3 minutes, flipping once, until nicely toasted on both sides. Remove from the heat but leave the broiler on.

On a rimmed baking sheet, place four big oven-safe dishes or crocks. Fill each bowl two-thirds full with hot soup. 1 piece of toasted bread, 2 slices of Gruyère cheese, and 1/4 cup

Asiago cheese should be placed in each bowl. Sprinkle a pinch of paprika on top of each one.

Cook under a high broiler for 5 minutes, or until bubbly and golden brown.

A beautiful melting crusty seal will form as the cheese melts and pours down the sides of the crock.

Enjoy and serve at the moment!

SWEET POTATOES, CARROTS, APPLES, AND RED LENTILS SOUP

INGREDIENTS

14 cup melted butter

2 big peeled and sliced sweet potatoes

3 big peeled and sliced carrots

1 peeled, cored, and chopped apple

1 chopped onion

12 c. red lentils

1 teaspoon sea salt

12 teaspoon fresh ginger, minced

12 teaspoon black pepper, ground

12 teaspoon cumin powder

12 tsp chili powder

12 tsp. paprika
veggie broth 4 cups

DIRECTIONS

In a big pot with a heavy bottom, melt the butter over medium-high heat.

Cook and stir sweet potatoes, carrots, apple, and onion for approximately ten minutes, or until onion is transparent.

After adding the liquid, whisk in the lentils, paprika, chili powder, ginger, pepper, and cumin. On high heat, bring the water to a boil. Once the lentils and vegetables are cooked, reduce the heat to medium-low, cover, and simmer for 30 minutes.

Using an immersion blender, puree the soup until it's smooth in the pot. After lowering the heat to medium-high.

simmer the sauce for ten minutes or so. As necessary, thin the soup with water to get the right consistency.

SOUP WITH BROCCOLI AND CHEDDAR

INGREDIENTS

3 teaspoons melted butter

14 tiny sliced onion

2 tbsp. all-purpose flour

1 cup sour cream

1 pound chicken broth

season with salt and black pepper to taste

2 cups broccoli, chopped

1 sliced carrot

1 sliced celery stalk

14 cup mild Cheddar cheese, shredded

DIRECTIONS

Melt butter in a stockpot over medium-high heat; add onion and sauté for 3 to 4 minutes, or until tender. Stir the flour in and whisk for an additional five minutes, or until golden brown.

Stir in half-and-half slowly until the onion mixture is smooth. Season with salt and ground black pepper to taste.

Reduce the heat to medium-low and continue to cook until the mixture thickens, about 10 minutes.

Mix in the broccoli, carrot, and celery. Simmer for 20 minutes, or until the veggies are soft but still crisp.

Turn the heat down low. Cook, stirring periodically, until the Cheddar cheese melts, about 5 minutes.

HEALTHY SUBSTITUTIONS TO MAKE DESSERT A GUILT-FREE TREAT

You can, indeed, have your cake and eat it, too. There's no need to dismiss dessert as a "bad-for-you" food. In fact, researchers contrasted eating dessert with breakfast when consuming less calories to not eating any dessert at all. During the "diet" period, both groups dropped nearly the same amount of weight. But here's where study gets interesting: once the dieting period was over, individuals who ate dessert with breakfast dropped an additional 15 pounds, while those who restricted sweets gained 22 pounds. To put it another way, you can have your cake and eat it, too. There are numerous healthy methods to satisfy your sugar tooth; all it takes is a little creativity and ingenuity. Everything you need to know about guilt-free

desserts is being broken down here, from easy ingredient substitutions to do-it-yourself recipes.

WHAT EXACTLY ARE "HEALTHY DESSERTS"?

Sweets that are reduced in sugar, suited to specific dietary needs (hello, gluten-free!) and prepared without (or with very little) artificial additives or hazardous fats are generally included. Other healthful ingredients, like dark chocolate and fruit, can also be included.

In fact, the perfect healthy dessert is a mix of the "Three Pleasures"nuts, fruit, and (dark) chocolate. For the over-21 population, a spirit-like port might be added as a fourth pleasure.

HEALTHY DESSERT RECIPES
It's no longer only buttercream frosting and hefty desserts. There are ways to make desserts fit into your lifestyle, no matter what your goals are, thanks to a
 wider availability of flexible ingredients and a deeper understanding of specific health demands, as well as cookbooks and blogs that specialize in these kinds of guilt-free desserts.

140

SUGAR SUBSTITUTES THAT AREN'T GUILTY

Trying to cut back on your sugar consumption? That doesn't mean you have to say goodbye to your favorite treats. There are several substitutes, but because sugar does more than simply provide sweetness it also leavens, browns, and drains moisture from components it's crucial to experiment until you discover the ideal substitute.

SUGAR MAPLE SYRUP

Its thick consistency is ideal for ice cream, pudding, and caramels. If the recipe calls for creaming, such as combining butter and sugar, you can substitute evaporated maple syrup, which comes in granule form like sugar.

HONEY

Honey has a comparable viscosity to maple syrup, although it dries out faster than refined sugar. It can be used in cookies, cakes, and fast breads. Because honey is sweeter than sugar, use a liberal 3/4 cup of honey for every cup of sugar. It also comes in a variety of tastes, so you may choose the flavor profile that suits your palate.

DATES

When creating almond milk (see below!), add a date to the blender, cut them up for brownies, or boil them down to a honey-like consistency to make date syrup. For every 1 cup of sugar, use 2/3 cup date syrup.

COCONUT SYRUP

Coconut sugar made from coconut flowers can enhance cookies, icing, and shortbread. It's a little on the dry side, so pair it with something wet, like mashed bananas or applesauce.

DIARY SUBSTITUTION FOR HEALTHY DESSERT
If you can't stomach dairy or just want to cut back, consider these milk substitutes:

ALMOND MILK

This alternative, considered one of the closest substitutes for dairy milk, has a creamy texture and a slight nutty flavor. And oat milk isn't just a terrific coffee creamer; it also works well in cakes, muffins, breads, and other baked goods. It is a 1:1 swap.

Milk from Almonds

You can use the same amount of almond milk as you would dairy milk, but because the former contains more water, your baked goods may rise and set faster. You may also wish to use a little sweetened version (rather than zero sugar) to match the natural sweetness of cow's milk.

SOY

Soy milk, which has a comparable protein profile to dairy milk, is a simple, mild-flavored substitute for dairy milk when you want to avoid nuts.

COCONUT CREAM

Is heavy cream called for in your recipe? Choose canned coconut milk, a nutritious, dairy-free alternative high in protein and satiating fat. When you open the lid, make sure to combine the thick cream on top with the more watery portion to achieve the desired consistency.

GLUTEN SUBSTITUTES FOR GUILT-FREE DESSERT

A new gluten-free flour league has created varied substitutes for refined flour. Keep in mind that if your recipe calls for all-purpose or wheat flour, using one of the gluten-free choices listed below may require some trial and error to obtain the desired texture:

ALMOND MEAL

This gluten-free choice is an easy substitution for all-purpose flour due to its mild flavor and 1:1 ratio.

COCONUT MEAL

It's popular as a low-carb alternative, but because it's so absorbent, watch your servings. In general, 1 cup of coconut flour

should be used for every 1 cup of conventional wheat flour.

CASSAVA STARCH

This gluten-free flour, made from the cassava plant's root, has a fine texture and nutty flavor that makes it ideal for breads, muffins, brownies, and pizza dough.

While many people refer to it as a 1:1 swap, because cassava flour is more absorbent, you should use less of it. You'll probably have to experiment with this one.

ARROWROOT
This cornstarch substitute, derived from the starches of numerous tropical fruits, can help thicken gluten-free dishes and form pastries.

SUPERFOOD SWAPS FOR GUILT-FREE DESSERTS

CHIA AND FLAXSEED MEAL

In addition to protein and fiber, these seeds are high in omega-3 fatty acids, which are essential for brain function. Make vanilla chia seed pudding and energy snacks with them. Another great option for replacing eggs is flaxseed meal.

CHOCOLATE (DARK)

The higher the cocoa percentage, the stronger the antioxidant properties (and the lower the sugar content). If you're baking brownies or chocolate chip cookies, use 70% cocoa or higher dark chocolate chips.

"SOFT BANANA SERVE"

There's no need for pints. For a potassium-rich alternative to ice cream and soft serve, combine frozen bananas with a splash of full-fat coconut milk.

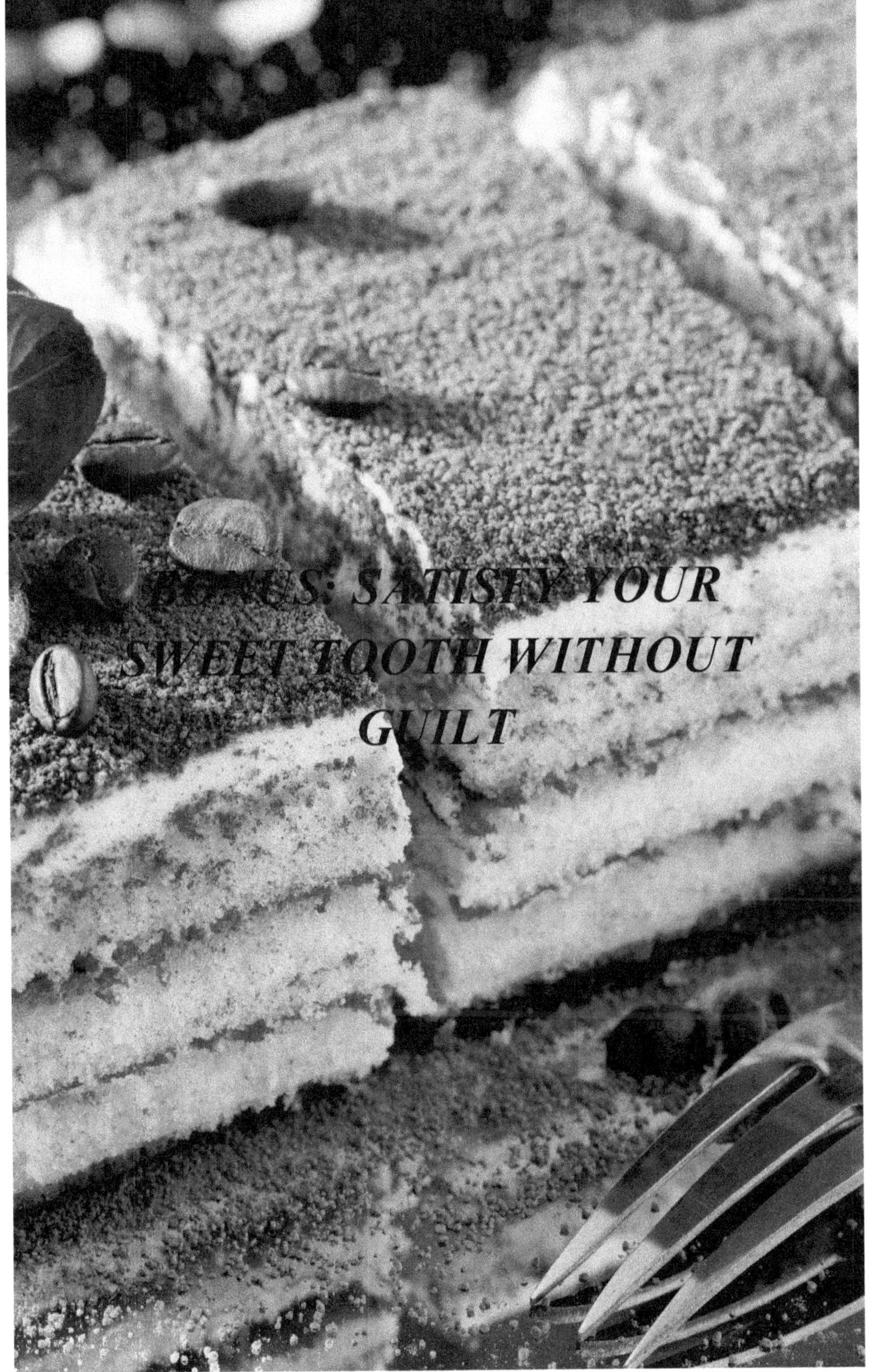
BONUS: SATISFY YOUR
SWEET TOOTH WITHOUT
GUILT

QUICK AND EASY HEALTHY DESSERTS

In a hurry and craving something sweet? These convenient guilt-free treats require little effort but deliver big flavor:

Chocolate-covered almonds, a dollop of peanut butter with cacao nibs, dates with dark chocolate, honey-drizzled fruit, and unsweetened coconut flakes.

HAVING SWEETS WITHOUT FEELING GUILTY

Instead of deprivation, you can make room for sweets in between all of those vegetable-focused, protein-packed, whole-grain-rich meals. The main thing is to make informed decisions. Rather than eating a sleeve of store-bought cookies, make your own healthier cookies with dark chocolate

chips and cacao nibs. Would you like something with a creamy texture?
Blend frozen bananas and garnish with sliced dates. If you need something quickly, keeping a few mainstays on hand peanut butter, chocolate-covered nuts, or dark chocolate pieces can be just the sweet, gratifying pick-me-up you require.

How to satisfy your sweet tooth without feeling guilty

12 delicious and indulgent, yet nearly guilt-free, goodies to create all year without violating your New Year's resolve.

RIPE PALEO CHERRY
This guilt-free cherry ripe, one of our favorite chocolate bars, contains only the best ingredients.

INGREDIENTS
2 1/2 cups dried cherries (375g)
Lemon Juice 100ml
1 tbsp additional honey, plus 1/3 cup (115g) honey
2/3 cup coconut oil (165ml)
1 cup shredded coconut (70g)
1 cup almond meal (100g)
3/4 cup cacao powder (75g), plus additional for dusting
1 cup (50g) toasted coconut flakes
1/2 cup (70g) roasted slivered almonds
1 tablespoon vanilla bean paste
30 halved and pitted fresh cherries

METHOD

1.In a saucepan over low heat, combine the dried cherries, lemon juice, 1/3 cup (115g) honey, and 1/3 cup (80ml) coconut oil, stirring constantly for 5 minutes, or until softened and melted. Add shredded coconut, almond meal, and 1/4 cup (25g) cacao to a food processor and whiz until mixed.

3.Transfer to a large mixing bowl and fold in the coconut flakes and slivered almonds.

4.Grease and line a 21 cm square baking sheet with baking paper, then press the mixture into it. Freeze for 2 hours, wrapped in plastic wrap.

5.In a small saucepan over low heat, combine the vanilla, extra 1 tbsp honey, remaining 1/3 cup (80ml) coconut oil, and 1/2 cup (50g) cacao to make a thick icing.

6.Cut into 15 bars with a heated knife. Dip the bars into the frosting and top with fresh cherry halves.

7.After 15 minutes, dust with additional cacao and serve.

POPSICLES WITH COCONUT, PINE, AND LIME

INGREDIENTS

2 x 400ml coconut milk cans

8 pomegranate

2 bananas, cut 2 mangoes, roughly chopped 1/2 pineapple, cored

2 limes juice

1 teaspoon turmeric powder

1 tablespoon rice malt syrup

1 tablespoon vanilla bean extract

2 tbsp non dairy milk (coconut milk)

METHOD

1. Shake the cans of coconut milk, then open and pour the coconut milk into three ice cube trays. Freeze for 24 hours.

2. Grease and line a 21 cm square cake pan with plastic wrap, leaving plenty of overhang on all sides.

3. Cut the passionfruit in half and scrape the flesh and seeds into a strainer set over a bowl, pressing down on the solids with a spoon to extract as much juice as possible. Remove seeds, saving juice.

4.In a food processor, combine the pineapple, banana, mango, passionfruit juice, lime juice, and turmeric until smooth.

Pour into the prepared pan and place in the freezer for 1-2 hours. In a food processor, blitz frozen coconut cubes, rice malt syrup, and vanilla for 4-5 minutes, in two batches, until smooth. (The mixture will get crumbly before it becomes smooth.

After 4 minutes, add milk to help the mixture come together.)

6.Pour over pineapple sorbet, insert paddle pop sticks at even intervals (the block will be sliced into 16 equal-sized squares), and freeze for 2 hours, or until firm but not rock rigid.

7.To serve, immerse the pan's base in hot water for a few seconds to soften the sorbet, then remove the block with plastic wrap.

Slice into 16 pops with a heated knife, then serve.

SLICED RASPBERRY, LEMON, AND COCONUT

INGREDIENTS

1 liter coconut oil

1/3 cup honey (115g)

1 1/4 cup almond meal (125g)

2 cups shredded coconut (140g)

2 lightly beaten egg whites

2 x 125g punnets halved raspberries

TOPPING
WITH COCONUT

2 tablespoons honey

1 gently beaten egg white

2 cups shredded coconut (140g)

CURD OF LEMON

3 eggs plus 3 more egg yolks

1 tablespoon cornflour, whisked with 1 tablespoon water

1/3 cup honey (115g)

2 lemons, finely grated zest and juice

1/3 cup coconut oil (80ml)

METHOD

1.Set or preheat the oven to 180 degrees Celsius. Line a deep 20cm 30cm baking dish with parchment paper.

2.Melt the coconut oil and honey in a skillet over low heat, stirring constantly. Combine almond meal, coconut, and a touch of salt in a mixing bowl.

3.Set aside for 10 minutes to cool before stirring in the egg whites until incorporated. Pour the mixture into the baking pan and press it down to form an equal layer. Bake for 17 minutes, until firm and brown. Place aside to cool.

4.To make the lemon curd, whisk together the eggs, egg yolks, and cornflour in a heatproof dish put over a pan of simmering water.

5.Continuously whisk in the honey, lemon zest, and juice for 4 minutes, or until thickened. Add the coconut oil and whisk for 4 minutes, until smooth. Set aside the curd to cool slightly.

6.Spread raspberries over the bottom. Chill for 1 hour to allow the lemon curd to solidify. Preheat the oven grill to medium heat.

7.To make the topping, melt the honey in a saucepan over low heat, then remove from heat. Whisk in the egg white until smooth, then fold in the coconut.

8.Spread the topping evenly over the lemon curd (don't flatten it because you want peaks of toasted shredded coconut), then grill for 2-3 minutes, or until the coconut is golden and crunchy.

9. Chill for 1 hour before cutting into serving portions.

BARS OF STRAWBERRY CHEESECAKE

INGREDIENTS

1 cup (135g) dates, soaked for 10 minutes in 1/3 cup (80ml) warm water

1 1/2 cups almond meal (150g) 1/2 cup desiccated coconut (45g), plus more to sprinkle

1 teaspoon cinnamon powder

1/4 cup cacao powder (25g)

1 tablespoon coconut oil

1/3 cup cacao nibs (40g), plus more to serve

To serve, sprinkle with coconut flakes.

METHOD

STEP 1: Grease and line a 23cm springform cake pan with parchment paper.

In a food processor, puree the dates and soaking liquid until smooth. Whiz in the almond meal, desiccated coconut, cinnamon, cacao, and coconut oil until barely blended. Pulse in the cacao nibs to blend.

3.Spread more desiccated coconut on the bottom of the pan, then add the date mixture and press into a compact layer. To set, place in the freezer for 20 minutes.

4.In a food processor with 1/4 cup (60ml) cold water, whiz all of the ingredients for 4 minutes, or until smooth, for the vanilla cheesecake. Return to the freezer for 2 hours to set after pouring over the base.

5.In a food processor, whiz all of the ingredients for the strawberry cheesecake for 4 minutes, or until smooth. (If the mixture is too thick, add 1-2 tablespoons of cold water; this will depend on the juiciness of the berries.) Return to the freezer for 3 hours to set after pouring over the vanilla layer.

6. 30 minutes before serving, remove the cheesecake from the freezer. To serve, cut into bars with a heated knife and sprinkle with cacao nibs and toasted coconut flakes.

BARS OF GINGER AND SESAME WITH A DRIZZLE OF PASSION FRUIT TAHINI

These ginger and sesame bars have all of the holiday flavor of gingerbread, plus some. They're also paleo, dairy-free, gluten-free, and high in fiber.

INGREDIENTS

2 grated carrots

LSA (linseed, sunflower, and almond meal) 1/2 cup (45g)

1 tablespoon ground cinnamon and ginger

1 teaspoon ground cloves and nutmeg

2 lightly beaten eggs

1/2 cup (180g) honey

1/2 cup (175g) ABC stands for almond, Brazil, and cashew. peanut butter

2 tablespoons coconut oil

1 tablespoon vanilla extract

1/2 lemon juice

2 tablespoons freshly grated ginger

1/2 cup (180g) roughly chopped pecans

1 cup toasted white sesame seeds

1 cup (70g) grated coconut

DRIZZLE WITH PASSIONFRUIT TAHINI

1/4 cup white tahini (70g)

2 tablespoons honey

four passionfruit

METHOD

1.Heat the oven to 180°C. Line a baking pan 18cm x 27cm with baking paper.

2.In a large mixing bowl, combine carrot, pecan, sesame seeds, coconut, LSA, and dried spices with a pinch of salt and powdered black pepper. Stir in the egg until well mixed.

3.In a small saucepan over low heat, add honey, nut butter, coconut oil, vanilla essence, lemon juice, and fresh ginger and cook, stirring, for 2 minutes, or until smooth and blended.

4.Pour wet ingredients over dry ingredients and mix to blend. Transfer the mixture to the prepared pan and smooth the top with a spatula.

5.Bake for 25 minutes, or until the center is set and the sides are caramelized.

6.Refrigerate for 2 hours to firm up after cooling to room temperature.

7.To make the tahini drizzle, mix the tahini, honey,

and 1/2 cup (125ml) water in a saucepan over low heat.

8.Stir for 2 minutes, or until smooth and melted. Take the pan off the heat.

9.Halve the passionfruit, then scoop the flesh, seeds, and juice into a mixing bowl and whisk to incorporate.

10. Allow to cool slightly before pouring over the bars and allowing to set before serving.

CHIA-CHOCOLATE BROWNIES

These all-natural brownies are topped with a gorgeous raspberry jam jelly and sweetened exclusively with dates and natural maple syrup. Cacao powder boosts antioxidant levels.

INGREDIENTS

20 pitted Medjool dates

1 tablespoon bicarbonate of soda

3/4 cup maple syrup (185ml)

3/4 cup (85g) unsalted butter, chopped cocoa powder

1/2 cup (80g) chia seed flour

3/4 cup (85g) shredded coconut

2 eggs

3 leaves of titanium-strength gelatine

375g raspberry chia jam or raspberry jam

METHOD

1.Set or preheat the oven's temperature to 160°C. Line a 20cm square baking dish with parchment paper.

2.In a saucepan put or place the dates and one cup (250ml) water. Place over medium heat and stir in the bicarb soda.

3.Bring to a simmer and cook for 10 minutes, stirring periodically, until thick. Allow to cool somewhat before transferring to a food processor.

4.Mix in the maple syrup and butter until smooth.

In a mixing dish, combine cacao, ground chia, coconut flour, and a pinch of salt. Fold in the date purée, then the eggs, one at a time.

6.Pour into a baking dish and bake for 25-30 minutes, or until set. Allow to cool completely in the pan.

7.To soften the gelatine leaves, soak them in cold water for 5 minutes. Heat the jam in a saucepan over medium heat for 2-3 minutes, stirring constantly.

8.Squeeze extra water from the gelatine and stir it into the jam.

9.Pour the jam mixture over the brownies and chill for 2 hours to solidify. Cut before serving into squares.

CHOCOLATE GELATO WITHOUT THE GUILT

The addition of yogurt to chocolate gelato gives it a nutritious twist. Probiotic-infused dessert!

INGREDIENTS

3/4 cup (165g) cane sugar

2 tsp corn flour 2 tsp sifted good-quality cocoa powder 375ml light evaporated milk

60g chopped dark chocolate

1 cup (280g) extra low-fat vanilla yogurt to serve

METHOD

1.In a saucepan, combine the caster sugar, cornflour, and cocoa powder. Mix in a bit of the evaporated milk to make a smooth paste. Stir in the remaining evaporated milk and simmer over low heat until the mixture thickens. Combine the dark chocolate and stir thoroughly until melted.
 and there is smoothness in the blend.
Remove from the fire and set aside for 15 minutes to cool.

2.Combine the chocolate mixture with the yogurt and chill for 30 minutes before pouring into a wide shallow container and freezing until the sides are frozen.

Remove from the freezer and whisk with an electric mixer. Go back into the container and re-freeze. Repeat 2 or 3 times, then place in the freezer for 4 hours, or until hard. (Alternatively, follow the instructions for an ice cream machine.)

3.Serve scoops of chocolate gelato with berry sorbet and, if desired, a dollop of low-fat yogurt.

PALEO PUMPKIN PIE

is the ultimate Thanksgiving dessert.

If you follow the Paleo diet, you will eliminate agricultural byproducts such as processed foods, refined oils, grains, legumes, and most dairy (please note that this dish uses butter). Try this simple pie to satisfy your sweet desire while staying within the Paleo diet.

INGREDIENTS

500g diced butternut pumpkin 600ml coconut milk

2 cup pecans (260g)

6 dates, dried

1 teaspoon vanilla essence, pure

50g melted grass-fed butter, cooled

1 tablespoon (35g) coconut flour

1 detached egg out of 3

2tablespoons cinnamon powder

1 teaspoon nutmeg, ground

1 teaspoon clove powder

1 teaspoon ginger powder

1/2 orange zest, finely grated

1/3 cup (80ml) maple syrup, with additional to serve
1/4 cup (40g) pepitas (pumpkin seeds)
To serve, coconut yogurt

METHOD
STEP 1: Preheat the oven to 180 degrees Celsius. Grease a 24 cm loose-bottomed tart pan with butter.

2. Stir pumpkin and coconut milk in a saucepan over medium-low heat for 25 minutes, or until soft. Cool.
3. In the meantime, blitz pecans and dates in a food processor until finely chopped, then combine with vanilla, butter, coconut flour, 1 egg white, and a pinch of salt in a mixing bowl.

In the prepared pan, press the mixture firmly into the bottom and sides. Prick the bottom with a fork and bake for 15-20 minutes, or until dry.

4.In a food processor, combine the cold pumpkin mixture, spices, zest, and 1/4 cup (60ml) maple syrup. Whiz together the remaining 2 eggs and yolk. Filling should be poured into the foundation. Bake for forty-five minutes, or just until the middle sets slightly.

5.Coat the pumpkin seeds with the remaining 1 tablespoon maple syrup.

Bake for 8-10 minutes on a baking sheet lined with parchment paper, or until brown. Allow to cool before breaking into shards.

6.Add yogurt, pumpkin seeds, and additional maple syrup to the top of the pie.

PALEO BANANA BREAD WITH PROTEIN

The nicest part about this recipe is that it makes guilt-free banana bread - the kind you can have for breakfast!

INGREDIENTS
Banana bread that is Paleo
three ripe bananas
1 cup (125ml) maple syrup, with more to serve
1 tablespoon vanilla bean paste
1 and half teaspoon ground cinnamon, plus additional for dusting
1 and half teaspoon bicarbonate of soda
12 cup (125ml) softened coconut oil
3 eggs
1 cup (110g) sifted coconut flour
1 cup almond meal (100g)
1 teaspoon baking powder
50g chopped pecans

METHOD

1.Preheat the oven to 160°C. Line a 1.5L loaf pan with baking paper and grease it.

2.Mash 2 bananas with maple syrup, vanilla, cinnamon, and bicarb soda in a mixing bowl. In a separate bowl, beat together eggs and coconut oil using an electric mixer.

In a mixing basin, combine the coconut flour, almond meal, and baking powder. Fold the banana mixture into the egg mixture, followed by the flour mixture and nuts.

3.Pour or Transfer the mixture into the baking dish. Cut the remaining banana in half horizontally and press into the batter. When the bread has baked for 55 minutes, a skewer inserted in the center or middle of the bread should come out clean.
Let the pan cool for half an hour.

4.To serve, drizzle with more warm maple syrup and dust with cinnamon.

BEACH BALLS MADE OF DATES AND NUTS

These small round bits of blended dried fruits, nuts, and seeds go well with coffee or as a quick snack.

INGREDIENTS

1 cup (100g) chopped walnuts, 2/3 cup (100g) chopped cashews, 100g blanched almonds, 1/2 cup (50g) chopped oats porridge instant

2/3 cup (100g) dried apricots, chopped

1/2 cup (150g) pitted dates, chopped prunes, pitted and cut

two tbsp sesame seeds

two tbsp cocoa powder

1 teaspoon cinnamon powder

2 teaspoons honey

1 cup (90g) coconut desiccation

METHOD

1.In a dry frypan over medium-low heat, toast the walnuts, cashews, and almonds for 2-3 minutes,stirring occasionally.

Place the ingredients in a food processor and pulse until finely chopped.

2.In a food processor, combine the oats, apricots, dates, prunes, sesame seeds, cocoa, cinnamon, and honey and whiz for 2-3 minutes, or until the mixture forms a paste.

3. Divide the mixture into 50g chunks (the size of a golf ball), then roll between lightly moistened hands to form around 15 balls.

4.Coat the balls in coconut before serving. For a maximum of two weeks, beach balls should be kept in an airtight container.

FINAL THOUGHT AND ENCOURAGEMENT

As you embark on this culinary adventure of fast, healthy, and tasty delights, remember that each recipe is a step towards a more flavorful and balanced lifestyle. Cooking doesn't have to be a chore; it can be a joyful exploration of tastes and a celebration of your well-being.

In the whirlwind of life, take a moment to savor the fruits of your labor, appreciating the vibrant colors and rich aromas that fill your kitchen. Embrace the simplicity of these recipes and let them be a reminder that nourishing your body need not be complicated, it can be a delightful experience.

As you dive into the world of swift and wholesome cooking, here are a few resources to further support your culinary journey:

Online Communities: Join forums and social media groups dedicated to fast, healthy cooking. Share your experiences, swap tips, and discover new recipes from a community of like-minded individuals.

Cooking Apps: Explore cooking apps that focus on quick and nutritious recipes. These apps often come with handy features like shopping lists, meal planners, and step-by-step instructions to simplify your culinary endeavors.

Cookbooks and Blogs: Expand your recipe repertoire by exploring cookbooks and blogs dedicated to fast, healthy cooking. Many authors and bloggers share their insights, experiences, and additional tips to enhance your culinary skills.

Local Farmers' Markets: Discover fresh, seasonal ingredients at your local farmers' market. Supporting local farmers not only adds a burst of flavor to your meals but also contributes to sustainable and community-oriented living.

Nutritional Guidance: Consult with nutritionists or dieticians who can offer personalized advice based on your dietary preferences and health goals. They can provide insights on how to make your meals even more tailored to your well-being

Remember, this journey is yours to personalize and enjoy. Whether you're a kitchen novice or a seasoned chef, the joy of cooking lies in the process. Embrace the adventure, savor the flavors, and nourish your body and soul with each delightful creation. Happy cooking!

Share Your Thoughts on "5 Ingredients or Less Plated Cookbook"!

Hi Reader's,

We hope you've been enjoying your culinary journey through the "5 ingredients or Less Plated Cookbook"! Your opinion matters a lot to us, and we would love to hear your thoughts on the book.

If you've found the recipes delightful, the flavors inspiring, or if there's anything specific that stood out to you, please consider leaving a review. Your feedback not only helps us understand what you loved about the book but also aids other readers in making informed choices.

Your insights are invaluable to us, and we appreciate you taking the time to share your thoughts. Thank you for being a part of our cookbook community!

Happy cooking!
Warm regards,
[Laura W. Gardner]